ballet-fit
workout

Published In the U.S. by
Ulysses Press
P.O. Box 3440
Berkeley, CA 94703
www.ulyssespress.com

First published in 2005 by ABC Books for the
Australian Broadcasting Corporation

ISBN 1-56975-438-1
Library of Congress Control Number 2004108853

Interior designed by saso content & design
Cover designed by Sarah Levin

10 9 8 7 6 5 4 3 2 1
Printed in Canada by Transcontinental Printing

Distributed in the United States by Publishers Group West

The exercises and advice given in this book are in no way intended as
a substitute for medical advice and guidance. Consult your doctor before
beginning this or any other exercise program. The Australian Ballet and
the Australian Broadcasting Corporation take no responsibility for any injury
that may be caused as a result of applying the information in this book.

ballet-fit
workout

develop strength, control, flexibility & grace

Megan Connelly
Paula Baird-Colt
David McAllister

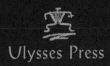

Ulysses Press

≫ CONTENTS

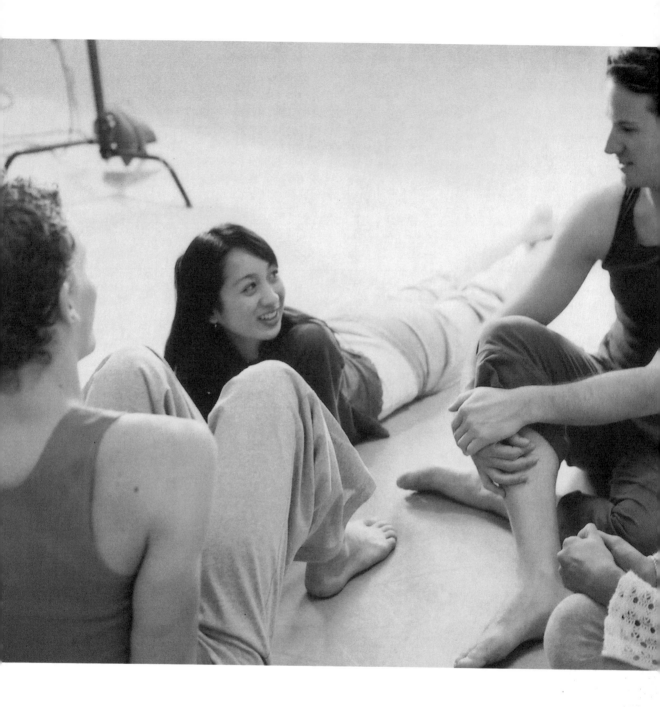

« ballet-fit workout »

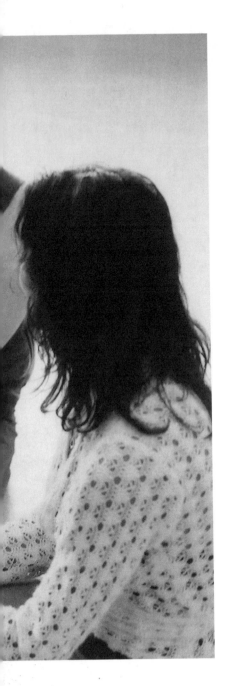

>> Foreword

Ballet dancers have captivated audiences for centuries with their effortless grace and physical beauty. Over time that physicality has changed and developed so that today's dancers are leaner and more athletic than ever before. They constantly push the boundaries of line and form and, in so doing, continue to redefine their technique and physical shape. But beyond their sheer physicality, dancers have a quality that sets them apart from other athletes: grace.

You can always spot a dancer in a crowd. Apart from the turned-out feet and generally oversize ballet bag, it is the regal posture, the elegant walk and a kind of glow that transcends the everyday. The truth is that most dancers don't even think about it. After years of meticulous training, a graceful poise becomes a dancer's norm, a subconscious discipline that is their natural bearing.

That is not to say that dancers don't think about the way they move. Their body is their instrument and every day, no matter how experienced they are, they reconnect with their body and refine their technique. This technique is not an end in itself—it is a means by which a dancer communicates abstract, narrative, contemporary, classical, dynamic or static ideas and movements. To do this successfully, dancers need an innate control and awareness of every fiber of their bodies.

While we can't hope to distill the many years of training required to become a dancer into one book, we would like to introduce you to some of the ideas and images that dancers use to help achieve their physical goals. It is our hope that you will be able to incorporate these movement principles and basic exercises into your daily life and exercise routine to help increase your awareness of your body and to achieve more grace!

David McAllister
Artistic Director, The Australian Ballet

>>the graceful

aligne

dynamic

rebal

awarene

holistic

body

>> The graceful body

The desire to move and to express ourselves through the body is innate. We all know that irresistible feeling when we spontaneously start moving to a special piece of music. You might have taken dance classes as a child or you might never have set foot inside a dance studio, but you still carry within you an ability to move expressively—you can dance.

Professional ballet dancers represent an elite group. They show us what can be achieved with a high degree of natural talent and years and years of dedication and training. But the purpose of this book is to demonstrate that there are certain principles that exist within the discipline of classical ballet that can be acquired by anyone who wishes to try. Their value is a more well-balanced, responsive and graceful body.

What are these movement principles? Essentially they are

alignment
dynamic stability
rebalancing
awareness
holistic balance

They are interconnected to the point of representing dynamic links in a chain of muscle, tendon, ligament, fascia, nerve and bone. By bringing about change in one link, you also influence all the others and create a smooth interplay between them that will make your body work better and feel better.

The body-conditioning program that we have devised will help you uncover your own elegance and grace. It will also enhance your body awareness and allow you to connect with your physical self with a new kind of mindfulness. Dancers have a highly attuned sense of their bodies that they nurture through repeated mind/body reconnections. By gaining a greater understanding of how you use your body, you will discover a greater sense of self and a greater connection with the environment. You will enjoy your body more. You will begin to move with the physical wisdom of a dancer.

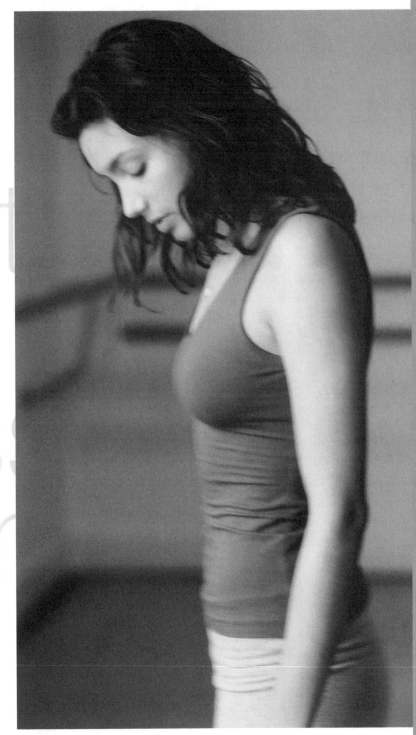

The most effective way to develop body awareness is to break movements down to their simplest form. We have selected our exercises for their simplicity, ease of learning and safety. They work in subtle but powerful ways to release surface tension and improve flexibility and alignment by allowing you to work with close attention to detail.

None of them are new. They are recycled and borrowed from Pilates, physiotherapy, the Alexander Technique, yoga and other methods. Where they may differ is in the primary focus, intention or cues within each one. They are designed to complement and refine whatever other exercise regimen you normally engage in. They provide a kind of secure base upon which you can build to improve your biomechanical efficiency in all your other activities.

Our program is suitable for just about everyone, including those people with limited physical ability or low levels of fitness. However, we suggest you consult a doctor before starting any new exercise program and please stop if you feel pain.

›› The key movement principles

Alignment

Well-balanced and efficient posture is the very foundation upon which all good movement technique is built. Postural work means developing a better understanding of how you place your bones, allowing your spine to support you naturally against gravity with minimum effort.

Dynamic stability

When the spine is lengthened and well aligned, the deep muscles that stabilize the pelvis and lower back activate naturally and provide support without tension. If you focus on rebalancing your spine each day, you will simultaneously improve the function of your deep musculature and develop better dynamic stability.

Rebalancing

Rebalancing is the process of finding neutral spinal and pelvic alignment. This applies to making regular reconnections as you go about your day as well as within the movements of each exercise. Focusing on a sense of symmetry in the placement of the bones and in muscular effort will help you rebalance your body. This in turn will help you to release unnecessary tension and develop smooth coordination.

Awareness

Begin to listen to your body. Notice how it is feeling and forge a closer relationship with your physical being. Rebalancing your body cannot begin until you recognize imbalances. This process is a journey of self-discovery that will enhance your life immeasurably.

Holistic balance

Our program encourages you to focus on your whole body and to bring all these movement principles together. The exercises take you through different parts of the body, giving you the opportunity to work on your center, your back, your lower body, your upper body and arms and your flexibility. The overarching intention is to provide you with the means of achieving the holistic balance that defines the graceful body.

Grace can afford us a lifetime of rewards and the good news is that there is more than a little bit in all of us.

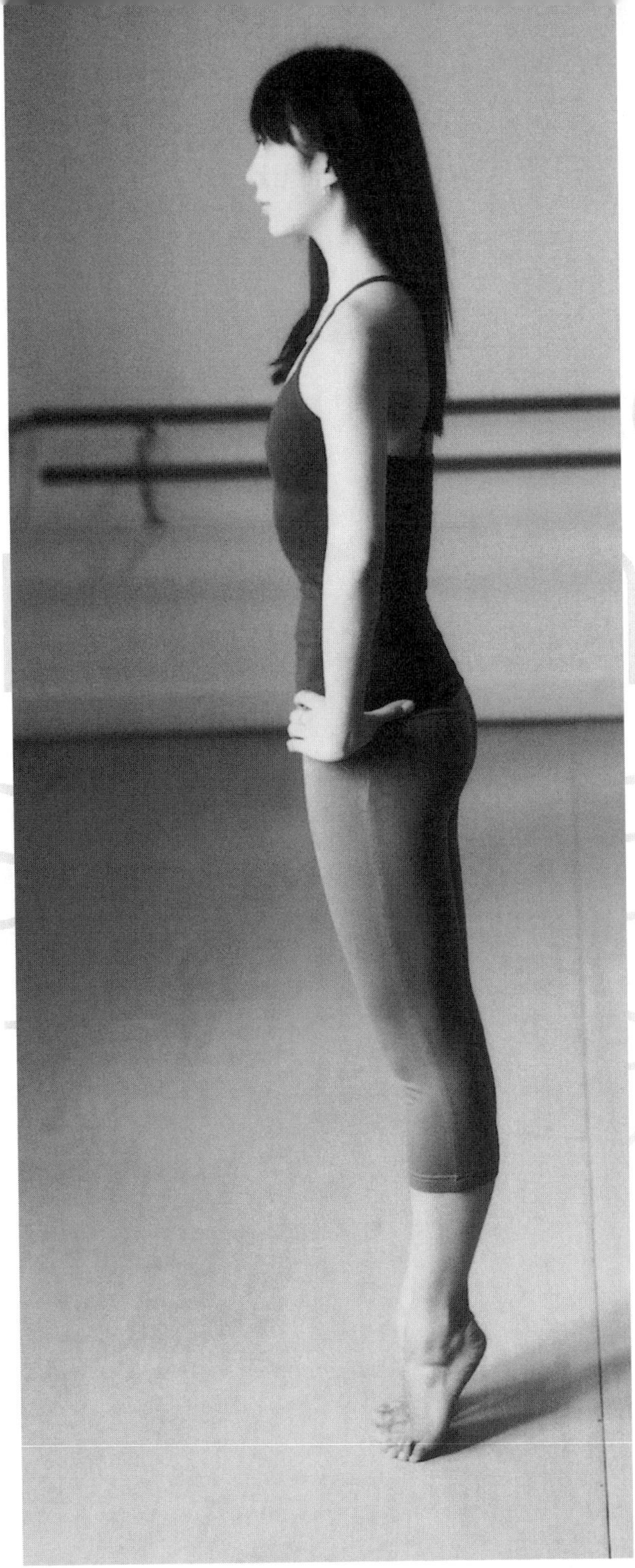

» Connecting body and mind

The body is an interconnected organism that functions best when all its parts are alive and responsive. Dancers aim to make each of their movements an organic, whole-body experience. Even when a movement appears to involve just one part of the body, a dancer will focus on how other parts respond at the same time.

The sensory information that is relayed from our muscles to our brains and back to our muscles via the central nervous system lets us know at any time where our bodies are placed in space. This circle of information is largely unconscious, allowing us to move around throughout the day without the undue distraction of worrying about our physical self. This is necessary, but it also means that many of us have a very poor awareness of habitual movement patterns, which ultimately does not serve us well. We simply don't realize when we are slumping or standing with all our weight on one leg or hunching with tense shoulders. Furthermore, because these movement patterns can be deeply ingrained they feel totally natural. They seem to be an inextricable part of who we are.

> # Live in your whole body, not just in your head.

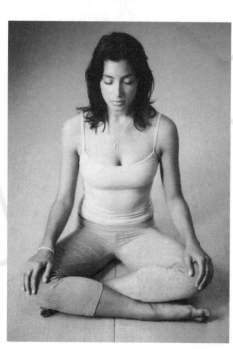

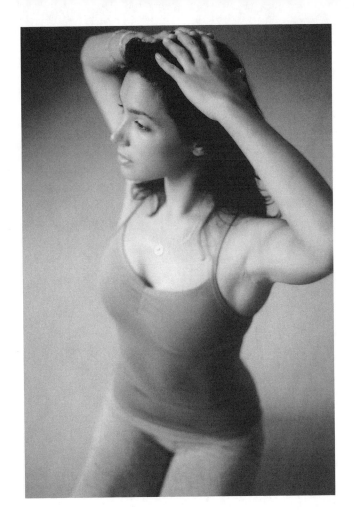

The exercises in our program can help you develop a better understanding of how you move and carry your body. They can be performed slowly, in your own time, and require you to think about and observe specific areas. This brings your focus to the way the various parts of the body feel when they are well placed and how they are interconnected with other parts. You will acquire a more organic sense of your body in space. Gradually this form of conscious awareness moves into your subconscious patterning and becomes integrated with how you move in your normal everyday activities. Over time you begin to replace your bad habits with movements that feature better biomechanical efficiency.

This process can be greatly assisted by using your breath. Bringing an awareness of your breath into an exercise helps you feel your whole body working in harmony. It collects body, mind and spirit together, releases tension and is wonderfully calming. Breath can be your best friend in developing movement flow and coordination.

This intimate connection between breath and movement helps to develop body synergy awareness. When you move freely and feel comfortable in your skin you will experience an enhanced joy of movement. You will know yourself better. But it does take time to change established patterns and discover new ones. Even dancers have to reconnect with their bodies daily to keep their awareness alive. Take the time to get to know your body and enjoy the freedom that it will give you.

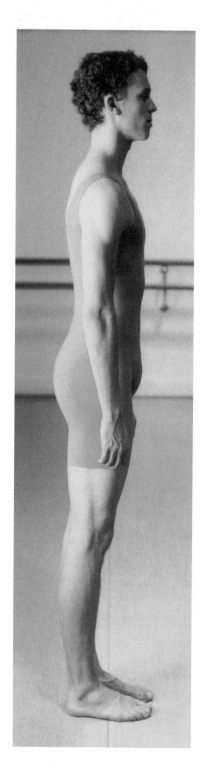

» The aligned body

It is easy to see how posture and alignment underpin every movement a dancer makes. Alignment is the quintessence of dance. The beauty of the line that the body sculpts in space is the purpose of each position that the dancer creates. On another level, alignment also plays a part in ease of movement and coordination. A well-balanced alignment leads to movement that feels better to the dancer and looks better to the audience.

Alignment is important for non-dancers as well. Not only does the body perform more efficiently when the entire body is correctly aligned, but there is also less risk of spinal pain, joint restriction and soft-tissue injuries. Good posture looks lovely and provides a way of moving with less strain and less muscle fatigue, allowing you more energy for everything else you do. Poor alignment, on the other hand, leads to surface muscle tension, incorrect muscle development, the establishment of incorrect movement patterns and pain, particularly in the lower back.

The principles of good alignment apply to any movement or environment. You will know you have started to improve when you recognize the way you hold your body at any given moment, whether you are performing a low-load activity, such as sitting, or something requiring much more skill, such as running, working out or dancing. It's a lifestyle check that will benefit you for the rest of your life.

Bony alignment

When we talk about alignment in our program, we are referring to the placement of the bones. The reason we do this is because it is easier to think about your bones than complex muscle actions. Optimal placement provides your muscles, ligaments and joints with the opportunity to work well. It allows you to adopt more sustainable movement patterns.

There are many other reasons why good alignment through the bones is beneficial to all of us, in addition to improving our general posture. A change in your alignment of just an inch or two, when you are working a specific body part, can take the impact of the exercise in a completely different area of the body from where you actually want it to be. If you work in poor alignment this strengthens the muscles that sustain that alignment. It is crucial that you pay close attention to your own posture in whatever type of activity you do, because it is the foundation of biomechanical efficiency.

Neutral spinal alignment

The spine is a complex structure that extends from the base of the skull to the base of the pelvis. It is made up of 24 separate bones, the vertebrae, plus the sacrum and the coccyx (commonly called the tailbone) at the base. The vertebrae surround and protect the spinal cord. Strong ligaments link them together and there is a flexible disc of cartilage between each one to absorb shock and to provide mobility.

Anatomists traditionally refer to the spine as having three curves, but dancers find it more functional to think in terms of four curves. They are in the neck (cervical), the upper back (thoracic), the lower back (lumbar) and the tailbone (sacral). It is important to respect these natural curves as they each perform a vital function. Try not to consciously flatten or straighten them into an unnatural alignment.

Start to improve your alignment by feeling a sense of length through the four curves and a connection through the vertebrae along a vertical line upward through the crown of the head and downward through the tailbone. This is neutral spinal alignment. It does not mean a single fixed position that you try to maintain, no matter what, because this works against your body's natural functioning. Rather, neutral spinal alignment is an optimal *zone* in which your spine feels lengthened and supported.

There are many moments throughout the day in which you can think about creating length in your body: sitting at your desk; sitting in the car; waiting for a train; walking down the street; washing the dishes; and getting some exercise. Let your imagination lengthen and move you!

» Dynamic stability

Dancers encourage dynamic stability when working with neutral spinal alignment. When the spine is lengthened and well aligned, the deep abdominal muscles that stabilize the pelvis and lower back—the transversus abdominis and the pelvic floor—are given the opportunity to activate naturally, providing stability at the center of the body.

The activity of these stabilizers allows us to let go of the surface muscle tension that can pull us out of shape. This is what we refer to in our program as dynamic stability: maintaining stability at the center of the body during movement, which allows us to recover and respond to the environment. *Dynamic stability* supports optimal placement and provides you with good functional posture through the total range of all your normal activities, both active and static.

We should move in and out of neutral spinal alignment all day as we bend, stretch, spiral and twist our bodies and this process is assisted by dynamic stability. Unfortunately, many people unknowingly perpetuate a negative cycle where poor body awareness and poor alignment contribute to weakness in the supporting muscles, which in turn contributes to poor alignment. For these muscles to work as they are designed to, they must be reawakened daily, otherwise they lose their capacity to respond. This can result in muscle imbalances as we unconsciously compensate by recruiting the larger external muscles to hold us up. The result is continued poor alignment, tension and pain.

You will start to improve your dynamic stability by noticing the alignment of your bones. Once they are in optimal alignment, most of the work is done. Bring your attention to your posture as you go about your day and remind yourself to place and notice the bones first, particularly the relationship between the spine and the pelvis.

Your center

We are almost never still. Our postural muscles are constantly engaged in supporting the spine and adjusting and maintaining our posture even when we are not consciously moving. It is not accurate to think of your center as something that "holds" you upright or "braces" you against gravity—this suggests something static and rigid. The muscular action is, in fact, more fluid and responsive. It is better to think of your center as being a ball of water that is always moving and working with and against gravity as required. The point is to think of it as alive and as a vital wellspring that creates energy in your body rather than consuming it.

Wear your body well

Neutral pelvic alignment

Imagine your pelvis is a shallow bowl filled with water. You must not let the water spill out the front or back of the bowl. Now visualize two horizontal lines: one running across the bottom of the bowl and one across the top. Keep your two sit bones on the bottom horizontal line and your two hips bones on the top line. We refer to this as neutral pelvic alignment. Our program will help you to combine *neutral pelvic alignment* with a lengthened spine, thereby improving your functional posture.

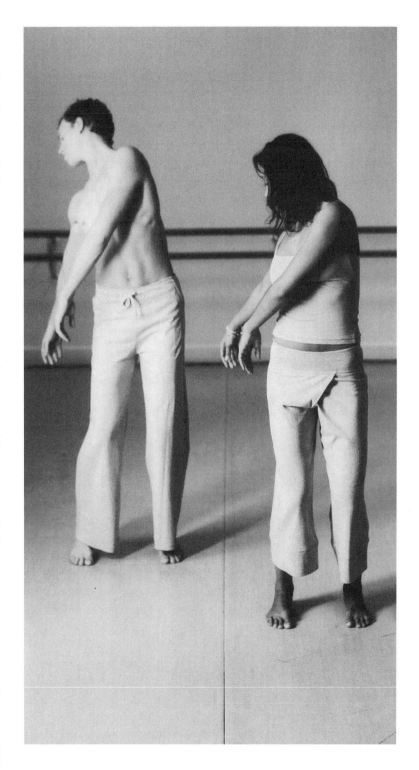

» Journey through the bones

Try taking a journey through your bones. Stand in front of a full-length mirror in your underwear or something tight fitting. Have a close look at the general shape of your posture and begin to identify some of the bony landmarks, working from the ground up.

Feet

Place the feet underneath the hip joints, about four to six inches apart, toes pointing forward. Make sure the second toe is pointing directly ahead of you. Feel the bottom of your big toe joint, little toe joint and center of the heel bone melting into the floor.

Knees

Let your knees soften, allowing them to absorb any imbalances in the legs and spine. Feel long at the front and back of your legs.

Sit bones and pelvis

Your sit bones should be pointing to the floor in a vertical line directly above your heel bones, with your center of gravity falling a little farther forward through the front of each ankle bone. This alignment helps keep the "pelvic bowl" balanced, without "spilling any water" out the front or back. You should now have a sense of the weight of the body being distributed through the three points of each foot. Keep the hip bones horizontally aligned, not twisted.

Spine

Lengthen the spine along a vertical line upward through the crown of the head and downward through the tailbone to the floor. Create space between the ears and shoulders.

Rib cage

Let the rib cage hang like a basket over the pelvis and feet.

Shoulders

Feel the tips of your collarbones and the bottommost tips of your shoulder blades broadening sideways.

Head

Align the ears over the sit bones.

Check the alignment of your body sideways in the mirror.

Now place your hands on your hip bones and begin to move your pelvis gently and slowly forward and back. Notice how playing around with the placement of your pelvis affects your posture as well as your height. You will be at your tallest in neutral spinal alignment. By exploring the connection between one part of the body and another, and how the placement of one part of the body affects another, you will begin to acquire good functional posture.

Find a moment to journey through the bones as often as you can to enhance your awareness of feeling your body in space. Enjoy the sensation of lightness and length that it brings.

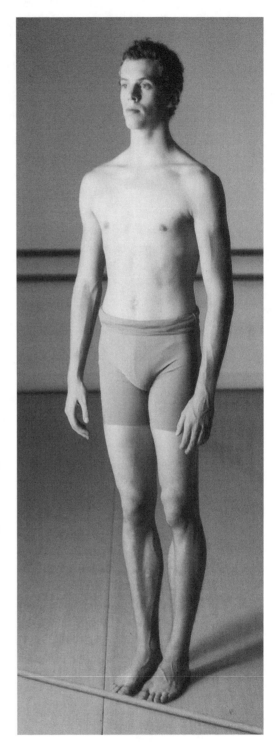

» Efficient abdominals

Efficient abdominals assist dynamic stability just as dynamic·stability assists alignment. This is not about developing prominent abs, because abs are the outer muscles, which do not play such an important role in maintaining alignment. Most people associate rippling abs with an athletic physique, but it's possible to have impressive outer definition with no dynamic stability. Rather, think about waking up your postural muscles each day by developing a sense of length and floating. Then you can forget about them and leave them to balance the forces on the spine. In this way you will not interfere with your natural patterning and your spine will find its most efficient balance without conscious effort.

It may be that you do not have sufficient endurance in these stabilizers to continuously support neutral spinal alignment. Dynamic stability is compromised if the underlying postural muscles are weak. In this case, you have to work slowly from the inside out, building endurance in the deepest muscles, the ones that are difficult to feel in the normal course of events, and gradually transfer this understanding to more intense movements. Your goal is to develop a sound base that will give you efficient abdominals that contribute dynamically to functional posture.

The deep unit

The deep unit comprises the transversus abdominis (TA), the multifidus and the pelvic floor. These are the deepest muscles in your center and the ones most implicated in good alignment. These exercises help you to discover and stimulate them.

TA and multifidus

These postural muscles support the spine with great natural endurance. They work close to the bones and often go unnoticed in daily activity. In the following exercise the movement sensations are small and subtle. Resist the temptation to overwork the muscles.

Kneel on all fours with a long neutral spine. Breathe in and let the belly relax and hang toward the floor. Breathe out as you very gently bring the belly button part of the way toward the spine. Try to maintain this connected feeling for up to ten natural breaths. You should experience a gentle stabilizing effect through your center, not a clenching sensation through the stomach muscles. The bones don't move during this exercise. Now release your belly button back toward the floor. Watch that your spine doesn't bend or flatten in the lower back as you do this.

The pelvic floor

The pelvic floor muscles are like a diamond-shaped hammock located at the base of the pelvis. You will wake up your pelvic floor by bringing the spine and pelvis into neutral alignment, but you have to reconnect daily with this deep stabilizer for this to happen. As with the TA, the action is deep and subtle, and this simple exercise helps you to become familiar with it.

In a sitting posture (see page 38), begin by identifying the four bony landmarks at each point of the diamond. The two sit bones mark the sides of the diamond, the pubic bone marks the front and the tailbone marks the back. You can find your sit bones by sitting on a firm chair and rolling the pelvis forward and backward—they're the ones you can feel digging into the chair. You can also sit on the back of your hands to help locate them. Gently draw the center of the diamond-shaped hammock upward and hold for up to 10 natural breaths in and out. If you lose the feeling of drawing upward during the ten breaths, just start again.

Monitoring of superficial abdominal muscles

When you encourage the use of the muscles of the deep unit be careful not to activate the more superficial muscles, such as the obliques and the "six-pack," unnecessarily. To monitor these muscles place your fingertips on your hip bones at the front and move them half an inch in toward your midline and press them half an inch into the muscle. Try this observational exercise to feel the difference between increased and decreased activity in the obliques. With your fingers pressed half an inch into the muscle, squeeze and grip all the abdominal muscles and feel the fingers being pushed out. Now release this activity and feel the muscles soften.

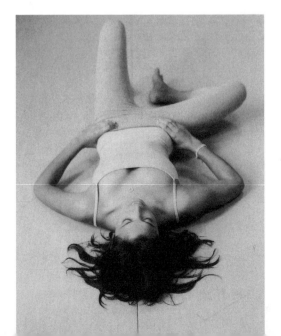

The best way to discover good functional posture is through exercise and movement because this develops your sense of how the whole body works as an interconnected whole. The process begins by finding ways to make daily mind/body reconnections and taking note of how your body feels. In addition to these exercises for the transversus abdominis, the multifidus and the pelvic floor, the observational exercises on pages 54 to 59 and the spinal wave exercises on pages 60 to 65 help you to discover the workings of your center and your own neutral spine alignment. You can perform them before you start a session or on their own at odd moments to refresh your body awareness. It's also highly effective to remind yourself to lengthen through the spine as you go about the day. This has the effect of awakening the postural muscles, making them more responsive and supportive.

›› Hips, legs and feet

Graceful, flowing movement and balanced alignment through the pelvis and spine are supported by healthy joints in the hips, legs and feet. If these become stiff, you may notice that your stride is shortened, making your walk tighter and more rigid. You free yourself up to move with relaxed grace when you mobilize your hips and you also improve your ability to support your alignment and keep your balance while performing a variety of dynamic activities, such as bending your knees and getting up again, stretching or climbing, as much as walking and running. The aim of the lower body exercises in our program is to help you develop healthy hips.

You probably know that classical ballet movements are based on *turnout*, or external rotation of the legs. This gives dancers a greater range of motion in the hips, a beautiful long line and a stable base on which to develop an acute sense of balance. Turnout may appear to come from the feet but it originates deep inside the hip. There is much debate within the profession as to which muscles are used or should be used by dancers to achieve the varied movements of the leg when they are externally rotated. As turnout is not essential for most of us, we present only simple and basic rotational work in our program. Nevertheless, your hips and legs will benefit from developing mobility in all directions.

You can begin by exploring the sensation of external rotation, first in the supine posture and then in the standing posture, with weight transfers. It is important to maintain neutral pelvic alignment during this work because this establishes a good relationship between the hip and the leg, which supports efficient functioning and ease of movement. Exercising the leg into inward rotation and in parallel alignment also mobilizes the hip joint and helps to correct muscle imbalances.

Pay close attention to our cues and images as you awaken a sense of isolation or independent movement in the limbs. Bringing your attention to this feeling is part of the process of connecting more deeply with your physical being and promoting holistic balance in your body. When standing in outward rotation, align the bones well with the knee on a vertical alignment with the second toe. Try to feel lengthened along the legs and through your spine. Keep the breath moving naturally.

Don't forget your feet. They are often neglected, so our program takes you all the way down to your toes and includes exercises and stretches to soothe aches and keep your toes flexible and strong.

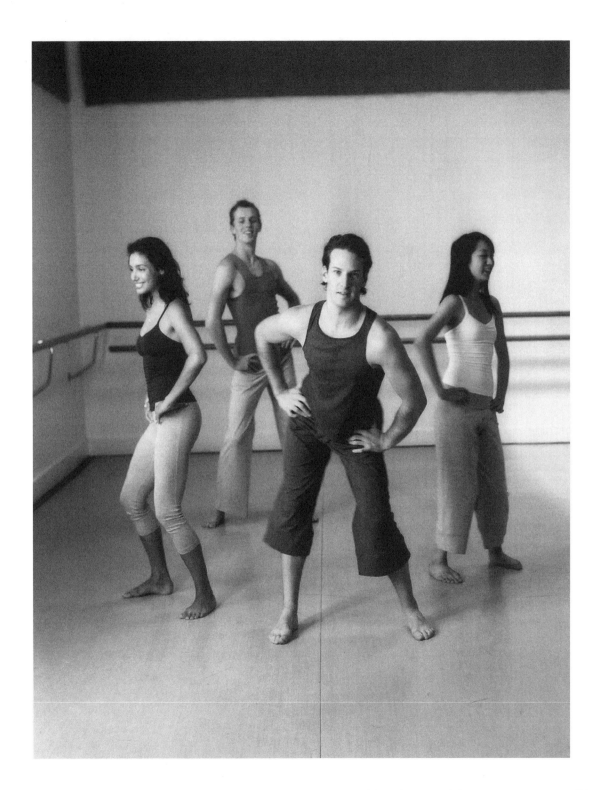

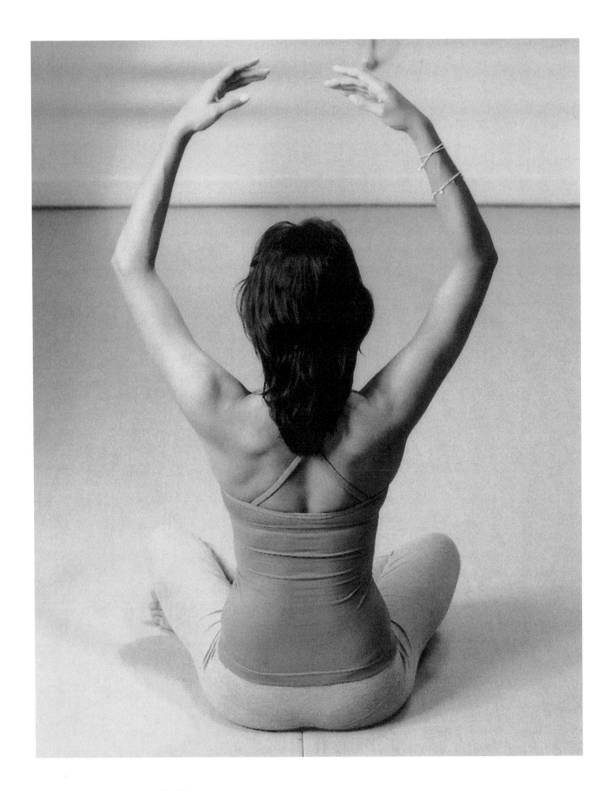

« ballet-fit workout »

» Upper back and arms

Much of the activity required to support functional posture occurs at the deepest level of skeletal muscle in a process that we rarely notice. But it is the carriage of the upper back, head and arms that conveys a distinctively attractive posture. This is the area of the body that clearly demonstrates grace and poise. It is mainly the movements and shapes of the upper body that create the difference between the many styles of dance as well as myriad emotions and moods that dancers are called upon to create. You could say that, in a wordless art form, dancers speak with their upper back, arms, hands and head movements. For the rest of us, developing elegance in this particular area leads to a more refined posture and better confidence in our bearing—which is perhaps the most important accessory to complement that little black dress or business suit!

Graceful posture relies on a sense of length through the spine and broadness across the upper back. Our exercises help to develop these qualities and promote mobility through the joints. The upper back and arm exercises focus on mobilizing the spine into flexion, extension and rotation. They also explore the relationship between the upper back and arms through the use of traditional classical ballet arm movements. Increasing the range of motion in all your joints gives your body healthy options to reduce and share loads and create ease in your movements.

Many of the exercises in our program are isolations of different movements to give you the chance to explore your range in certain areas like the shoulder joint. Take full advantage of your arm range to reduce unhealthy patterning and to stay light and free in your movements.

Tension inhibits flow. A tight neck affects the entire upper body, so we have included exercises to help you release unnecessary tension. Remember that the neck is part of the spine and should feel lengthened along the same vertical line. Keeping your eyes focused directly ahead helps to maintain the alignment of the neck. This does not just apply to when you are exercising, but to many everyday situations. For example, if your computer screen is below your eye level, you are more likely to hunch over into poor postural alignment.

Whenever you can, use the imagery from the upper back exercises in our program to help you develop a graceful confidence in your posture.

>> Flexibility

The one activity that dancers engage in repeatedly that even very fit non-dancers rarely do frequently enough is stretching. Their flexibility means that they can move smoothly in and out of positions with an effortless grace and sensuous beauty. This is the product of moving through their full range from an early age. For most people, stretching is something they do for a few short minutes at the end of a workout. And some people never stretch.

Active and conscious stretching is an important part of maintaining good health throughout life. It offers many benefits, such as improving range of motion, releasing tension and rebalancing the body. People often think only of lengthening muscles when they think about flexibility, but it is also about moving a joint through its full, normal range of motion. We strongly recommend that you gently mobilize joints before exercising, and we include effective mobilizing exercises in our program for the arms, hips and legs and back to include in your warm-up. This is important for keeping connective tissue nourished and maintaining quality of movement.

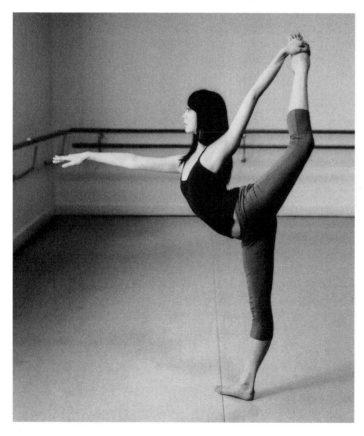

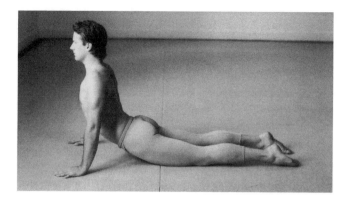

Furthermore, better flexibility in places where you are particularly tight, such as in your hips or between your shoulder blades, improves your alignment and make it easier to organize your bones correctly. However, alignment is also essential for a stretch to be safe and beneficial and this is where attention to detail is crucial. If the body is not aligned then you perpetuate muscle imbalances, thereby reinforcing a negative cycle. By keeping the bones well aligned while you stretch, you reinforce a positive cycle in which flexibility improves alignment and alignment improves flexibility.

We all have different degrees of natural flexibility and frequently one side of the body is tighter than the other. Bring your full attention to each stretch and, without making any judgments about your ability, observe your own areas of tightness. This helps you to build your internal picture of your body. Breathe evenly, releasing all the air with each exhalation, to let go of tension and to make the stretch a vital, whole-body experience. It might be uncomfortable if you are unused to it and have stiff, tense muscles, but working them gently will leave you feeling relaxed and centered.

Remember that our bodies have a huge capacity for suppleness and movement and that as soon as you start to stretch you free yourself up to move more naturally.

Notice that some exercises are followed by suggested stretches from the "Lengthen and Release" section, which you may find beneficial to do.

There are various stretching techniques, but in our body conditioning program we use two different ways to safely maximize your flexibility: joint mobilization and sustained stretching. We recommend that you use joint mobilization as part of your warm-up phase, accessing your existing range of movement. Sustained stretching of muscles is more beneficial in your cool-down phase to further increase your range of movement when you have elevated your core temperature and your joints and muscles are warm with good blood flow.

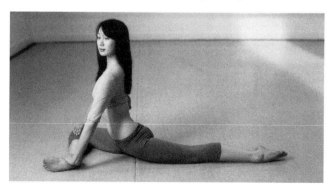

›› Overcoming movement habits

A good movement technique should free you. It should not bind, exhaust and deform the natural balance that exists deep inside all of us. However, most people have developed multiple bad movement habits in the course of their life and have little or no understanding of their body's intuitive natural balance.

When we learn a movement pattern, the brain sets up a neurological pathway in the central nervous system. This applies to the huge range of physical activities in which we engage each day, both the mundane and the specialized, starting with the action of getting out of bed in the morning. If we continue to perform movement patterns in the same way, then the neurological pathway becomes firmly entrenched and habitual. We're usually unconscious of this process. We don't realize that the way we move is due to the force of habit: it's just the way we move.

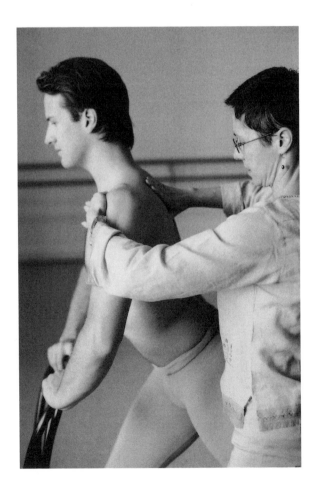

The great difficulty to overcome is that bad habits feel completely natural and balanced when they are not, even if they cause discomfort. If you habitually slump when you sit at the computer each day, then that is your normal way to sit. When you attempt to sit with good alignment, it will feel unnatural and uncomfortable. Your neuromuscular system will keep on returning to its habitual mode and you'll find you've slumped again.

You can replace your bad movement habits, but for this to happen you have to work steadily on your awareness, so that you can disrupt automatic, unconscious ways of doing things. By consistent daily reconnections with your body, you encourage it to respond differently and to find a more balanced way to maintain a lengthened alignment. As this gradually improves, so better dynamic stability and coordination will begin to follow. Eventually, more efficient patterns that benefit your body will become dominant.

It may help to bear in mind that what you are doing is not learning new ways of using your body so much as rediscovering ways that you once knew when you were very young. Children learn to stand and move with an intuitive sense of alignment. Eventually, these natural patterns can become overlaid with a variety of careless habits caused by a host of factors including stress, weak muscles, accidents or injuries, a negative self-image, inactivity. Be assured that the understandings you need to make changes are within your body memory and can be reanimated with time and attention to detail.

Performing the exercises in our program gives you a dedicated time to focus on your body and become acquainted with its abilities and limitations. To stay mindful of what you are doing and alert to your physical responses, don't always start them with the same leg or perform them in the same order.

As you do our exercises and experiment with new approaches to movement, remember that it's all about the process, not the goals. Indulge in the exploration of movement and let go of old movement patterns so that you can find freedom in your posture and alignment. Allow yourself to "fall over" just like babies do when they first learn to stand. You'll only learn something new by falling over a few times!

Use everyday situations as opportunities for increased body awareness. Stand tall in the supermarket queue, stretch and extend your spine in your chair at work, focus on your breath when you are running late, swing your hip bones around while you are doing the dishes. These are all times to enjoy your body and to simply be in it.

›› Letting go of tension

Pain and tension are enemies of good movement patterning and smooth coordination, and you have to become aware of their effect on the body before you can fully overcome poor movement habits. Poor alignment causes tension and tightness. Muscle imbalances can cause aching in the lower back or tightness in the shoulders and neck. Unfortunately, holding muscular tension in certain parts of your body can once again become habitual and unconscious. Often we tense up because of stress, but if we don't learn to let go then our bodies never fully relax and return to a state of ease.

As you journey through the bones, observe where you tend to hold tension. Perhaps you grip your buttocks or pull your knees up tight or clench your jaw. Quietly let go and feel the muscles soften. When you perform the exercises, be aware of tension creeping in. As you work on one part of the body, make sure that you are not gripping elsewhere. It is counter-productive to hold yourself tightly in an effort to "work harder." This disrupts holistic balance and coordination and interferes with sensitivity to fine adjustments in a movement—not to mention making the exercises much less enjoyable to do.

With awareness, letting go becomes easier with each attempt.

Unlearning tension can be a difficult process, in the same way that it takes time and persistence to retrain your movement patterns. Nevertheless, a release technique can be as simple as becoming aware of your breathing. You can often release tension from your jaw, neck and shoulders simply by breathing out and this is a useful thing to remember throughout the day.

Exercise itself can help you relax. As you concentrate fully on your physical self, your mind calms down and tensions from everyday life recede. Your session should leave you feeling refreshed, deeply satisfied and returned to yourself.

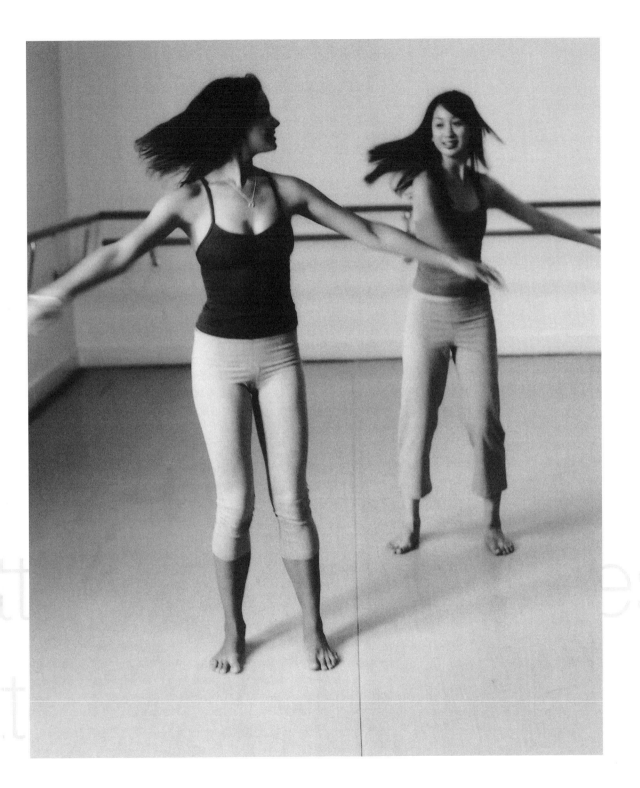

» Breathing

Just as many of us are not mindful of how our bodies are placed at any given time, so we do not give a great deal of attention to our breath. Breathing is an instinctive and involuntary process, but the combination of stress, holding muscular tension and poor alignment can restrict the natural flow of our breath in the same way as they restrict our natural freedom of movement.

By coordinating your breath with movement you help your body find its natural patterning and develop a holistic balance. Breathing well also helps you to release unnecessary tension. As your body awareness grows, you realize when you are tensing up and you can send your breath deeply into your body to help you to let go.

If you consciously bring an awareness of your breath into an exercise, you generate a sense of the whole body working in harmony. With regular practice and attention you find that your breathing becomes easier and more naturally integrated with the movements.

We have not given many breathing cues in our exercise descriptions. Generally, we believe it is best for you to find your own natural rhythm and to be aware of the changes in your breathing patterns during the movements in each exercise. Play around with the timing of the inhalation and exhalation to find out what suits you best for each particular movement. Be careful not to exaggerate the breathing because this can make you use certain muscles unnecessarily. Focus on bringing the breath movement into the side of the ribs instead of the front of the ribs or into the stomach. The observational exercises on pages 54 to 59 help you become aware of your breathing. When you have become familiar with each one, we recommend that you do the exercise "breathing sideways into the ribs with awareness" on page 58 before you start an exercise session.

» Imagery

Language is an immensely powerful tool. Because all words contain a complex, personal history of subconscious associations, it's vital that you use productive terms with yourself as you seek to improve your alignment or when you practice any of our exercises.

When certain words are used as cues or instructions they can have the unfortunate effect of increasing surface muscle tension and impairing movement. Terms such as "brace" or "hold" tend to make dancers grip or tighten their external muscles and this restricts their full range of movement. On the other hand, terms such as "lengthen" or "float" help them to release tension and open their bodies to move with more ease and grace.

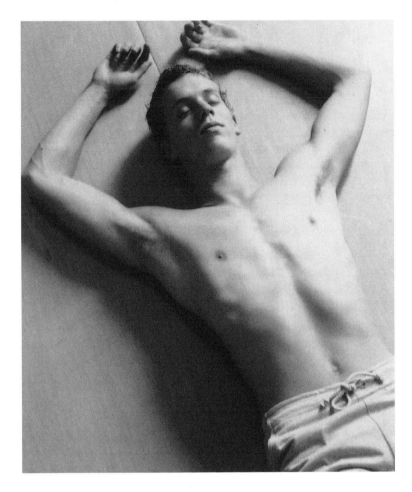

Occasionally telling yourself to pull in your stomach will not help you strengthen your abdomen. It's more likely to encourage you to recruit the internal and external obliques for a short while. These muscles are not designed for that and they will quickly fatigue and you will be back where you started. But if you tell yourself to balance your pelvis like a bowl of water you will awaken the deep stabilizing muscles that support the spine.

Pay attention to the verbal cues that we have provided in the exercises because we've chosen each word deliberately to help you perform the movements with biomechanical efficiency. Listen also to your self-dialogue. It is counter-productive to tell yourself to work harder or to pull or squeeze or any similar term. Instead, use the images we suggest and reassure yourself that the exercises are about exploration and discovery. You cannot force your body to become more free-flowing: it knows how to find it once you let go. Focus on the process, because this leads ultimately to greater rewards.

›› Injury prevention and rehabilitation

Injury-prevention programs have become a large part of a dancer's life, to guard against the often extreme and complex movements created by today's choreographers. Dancers try to identify their underlying physical weaknesses and imbalances and address them with a simple but intense program of exercises. The exercises here are designed according to the same principle. They are simple enough to be easy to understand and perform with close attention to detail but intense enough to be highly effective in helping you to rebalance your body and guard against injury.

Dancers have a well-honed body awareness that helps them listen to their body, notice changes such as muscle tightness and stiffness and respond accordingly to prevent injury. As you develop your own body awareness you may find that you are feeling tighter or weaker than usual in one area—for example, your shoulders and upper back after you've spent the weekend moving furniture or your hamstrings while training for a fun run—and you can use our exercises to focus on that problem for a while, until it is relieved. This will help you to protect yourself against possible future injury and puts our program to good use.

Of course the most basic injury prevention rule is warming up and cooling down before and after exercise. Always begin an exercise session by raising your core body temperature and mobilizing the joints. Complete a session with general all-body stretches or, at the very least, stretch out those areas that have been worked.

Rehabilitating after an injury can provide you with an excellent opportunity to improve movement habits and realign the body. In fact, many dancers find they are in better condition after an injury than before. Depending on the injury, the exercises in our program can be used as an effective part of any rehabilitation program. Dancers use various programs and techniques to rehabilitate, including working in the weightless environment of a swimming pool. But remember, prevention is always best. Making a commitment to improving your functional posture by rebalancing your body every day will help your body to become more resilient and less prone to muscle fatigue, tension and injury.

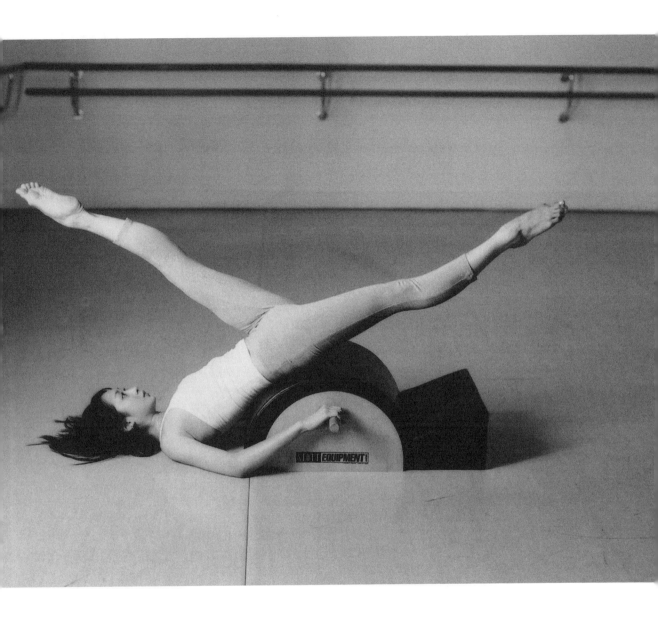

» Cross-training

Research and development in the area of dance medicine over the past 20 years has educated a generation of dancers and dance teachers about a more scientific approach to classical ballet technique. This knowledge has led to a better understanding of injury-prevention methods as well as the benefits of cross-training. One of the most important benefits of this knowledge is assisting ballet dancers to strike a balance between the aesthetic demands of classical ballet and muscle durability and strength. For example, Pilates and yoga offer dancers alternative methods of discovering alignment and "release" techniques to help prevent repetitive strain injuries. Swimming and cycling improve cardiovascular fitness and breath control. These different exercise regimes are also a necessary part of rehabilitation programs for dancers recovering from injury.

Not surprisingly, cross-training benefits the non-dancer as well. It's perfectly natural to continue to engage in an exercise activity that you enjoy, but as your body adapts to it you are less likely to notice further improvement, particularly if you repeat the same work at the same level of intensity each time. If you vary your regime by taking part in more than one kind of activity, you give your body the chance to move and explore through a greater range of neuromuscular challenges. This develops your versatility and stimulates your coordination, as well as making life more interesting. Just make sure you check with your doctor if you have any concerns about your health or fitness, then find a professional instructor for the best advice on your chosen activity.

Our program is intended as a basis for aligned, functional movement and prepares you for any kind of exercise. It doesn't matter if you prefer sports or yoga, or if you love strength training or running in marathons: you need a full understanding of your own posture in a full spectrum of dynamic applications to protect yourself from injury and to perform with biomechanical efficiency. Use our exercises to complement your favorite activities and enjoy the rewards.

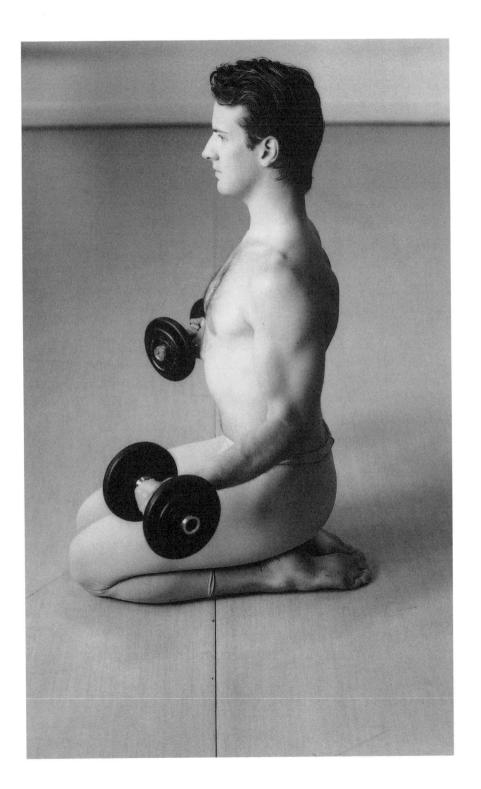

» From start to finish

It is important when exercising to be safe and comfortable. You don't need to be anywhere fancy—exercising on the rug in the living room is just as good as on the floor at the gym. Just make sure you are not working on a cold surface, such as concrete, or in a drafty area.

You may feel more comfortable using an exercise mat, depending on where you are practicing. These are usually inexpensive and can be found at sports stores—even camping stores have thin rubber mattresses that can serve as exercise mats. Some of our exercises use basic equipment: a chair or ball, a thin broomstick and a towel or elastic exercise band.

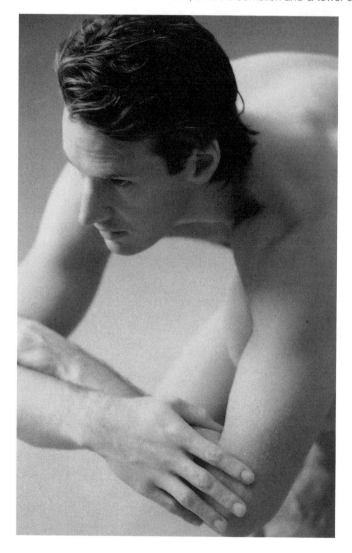

Warming up

Take between five and 15 minutes to warm up with some aerobic work at the beginning of each exercise session to give you a more effective workout and prevent injury. A good warm-up can be as simple as walking, jogging, cycling or mini-trampoline jogging until your heart rate has increased and you have begun to break into a sweat. This activity will get the blood flowing to the muscles, making them pliable and ready for the work ahead.

Choose your preferred warm-up exercise and gradually build up to 15 minutes of aerobic work before each session—you will gradually increase your fitness level too! Remember to wear supportive and comfortable footwear and try to avoid hard surfaces.

Cooling down

Cooling down immediately after exercise is a vital component of injury prevention and muscle recovery and helps reduce muscle stiffness and soreness. This can be as simple as going for a walk. Depending on how strenuous your workout was, it is beneficial to do between five and 15 minutes of mild exercise to cool down.

The next part of the cool-down phase is stretching. When you have finished exercising, it's a good time to work into the stretches and develop your flexibility. Make sure you stretch the muscle groups that were worked during the exercise program. It's also a good time to drink some water to replace any fluids lost through perspiration.

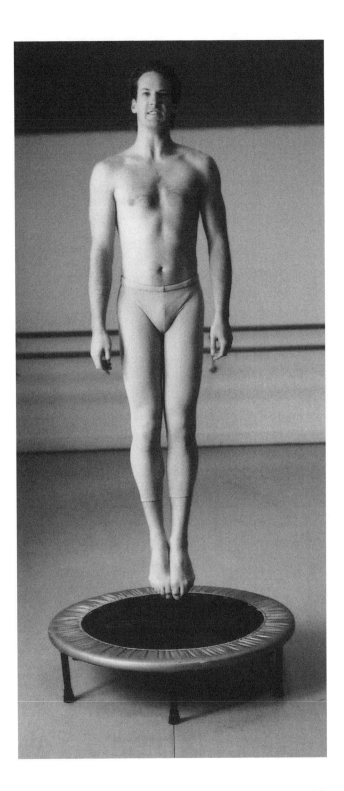

» What to wear

It is best to wear close-fitting clothes that make it easier to see your posture and alignment, and fabrics that feel comfortable and stretch well, so that they move easily with your body. Remember to wear fabrics that breathe to allow any sweat to evaporate, particularly during aerobic exercise. Everyone has an individual style and it is important to wear exercise clothes that you like.

While dancers wear an assortment of shoes from the iconic pointe shoe to heeled boots when they're dancing, it is best to do the exercises in our program either in bare feet or wearing socks. You can try both (as long as you're in a warm environment) because they give you very different sensations and connections to the floor.

Our exercises encourage you to release tension while you work—if you have long hair let it out.

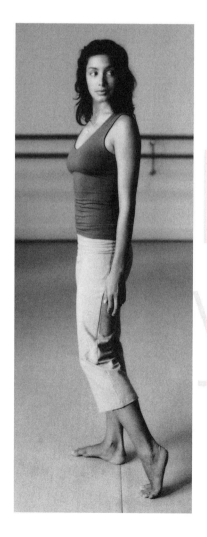

If you feel good, you will exercise well.

» What to listen to

Music plays a vital role in a dancer's life. It is the canvas on which the steps sit. More often than not, a choreographer uses music as a starting point when creating a new work. He or she finds inspiration in the drama or flow of a particular composition and translates it into movement.

In the studio, music can affect the execution of an exercise through the use of different rhythms and dynamics. Our exercises rely more on an internal rhythm than music, but whether or not to listen to anything is up to you. We have included a selection of music that may enhance your workout and assist you in the experience of truly connecting with your body.

ROMEO AND JULIET
Sergei Prokofiev
Recommended recording:
Valery Gergiev, Kirov Orchestra,
Philips, 432166

SLEEPING BEAUTY
Pyotr Il'yich Tchaikovsky
Recommended recording:
Mikhail Pletnev,
Russian National Orchestra, DG

SERENADE FOR STRINGS IN C
Pyotr Il'yich Tchaikovsky
Recommended recording:
Orpheus Chamber Orchestra,
Polygram, 423060-2GH

THE NUTCRACKER
Pyotr Il'yich Tchaikovsky
Recommended recording:
Antal Dorati, the Royal
Concertgebouw Orchestra,
Philips 464747

GISELLE
Adolphe Adam
Recommended recording:
Andrew Mogrelia, Slovak Radio
Orchestra, Naxos 8.550755-56

PRELUDE A L'APRES-MIDI
D'UN FAUNE
Claude Debussy
Recommended recording:
Bernard Haitink, the Royal
Concertgebouw Orchestra,
Philips, 464697-2

LE SACRE DU PRINTEMPS
Igor Stravinsky
Recommended recording:
Bernard Haitink, London
Philharmonic Orchestra, Philips
2894383502

SCHEHEREZADE
Nicolai Rimsky-Korsakov
Recommended recording:
Eugene Ormandy, Philadelphia
Orchestra, Legacy/Sony Classical
089956

MIDSUMMER NIGHT'S DREAM
Felix Mendelssohn-Bartholdy
Recommended recording:
Philippe Herreweghe,
Champs Elysees Orchestra,
Harmonia Mundi 9488130212

SYMPHONY IN C
Georges Bizet
Recommended recording:
Sir Neville Marriner, The Academy
of St. Martin in the Fields,
EMI 2435737092

APOLLON MUSAGETE
Igor Stravinsky
Recommended recording:
Igor Markevitch, London Symphony
Orchestra, Philips 2894383502

SWAN LAKE
Pyotr Il'yich Tchaikovsky
Recommended recording:
Richard Bonynge,
The National Philharmonic,
Decca 473283-2 DF 2

DON QUIXOTE
Leon Minkus
Recommended recording:
Nayden Todorov, Sofia National
Opera Orchestra, Naxos
8557065-66

» Using the program

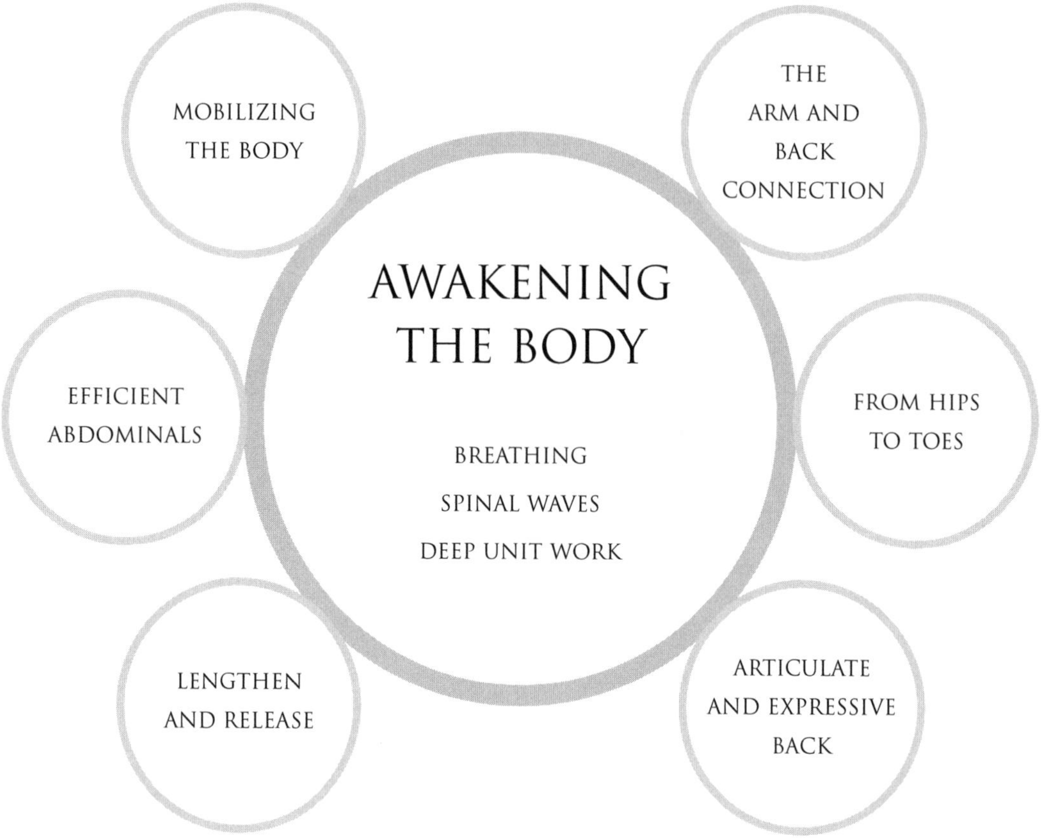

MOBILIZING
THE BODY

THE
ARM AND
BACK
CONNECTION

EFFICIENT
ABDOMINALS

AWAKENING
THE BODY

BREATHING

SPINAL WAVES

DEEP UNIT WORK

FROM HIPS
TO TOES

LENGTHEN
AND RELEASE

ARTICULATE
AND EXPRESSIVE
BACK

It is best to think of our body-conditioning program as a circle.

The observational breath exercises, the spinal wave exercises and the deep unit work in the section "Awakening the Body" form the central focus of the work and link all the different areas together. They can be done anywhere, anytime. We suggest you begin by familiarizing yourself with them before moving on to other areas of the program. For some of you, this may take 15 to 20 minutes a day for a week or two; others may find they require less time.

Try to find time to reconnect with your body daily. This will take less and less time the more consistently you do so. Remember to take these reconnections into your day with you.

When you are ready to move on, choose a spinal wave in one of the essential postures (supine, sitting or standing) with which to start and finish each exercise session. Choose a different posture every few sessions. Include also the breathing exercise "breathing sideways into the ribs with awareness" on page 58.

Then it's time to try the various mobilization exercises for the arms, hips, legs and back. Explore your range of movement in the major joints of your body and discover your areas of stiffness and vulnerability. Become familiar with these exercises because they form part of your routine warm-up. Once you have warmed up, you are ready to move on to the other exercises.

Refer to the program circle to decide how you wish to proceed. You may choose to fully explore one section, such as the arm and back connection, and exclusively follow this program for a few days. Or you may choose to do one exercise from each section and work through the entire body. Or you may want to select different exercises for just the one area of your body that's feeling particularly stiff or tense.

Play around with the order to keep your brain guessing, which will help avoid slipping into habits. Whatever you choose to do, it's important to alternate between sitting, standing and lying postures. This keeps you moving and highlights the essential fact that good functional posture is not an immovable, single position: it is a zone we move in and out of during everything we do, every day.

Remember to cool down with some stretches from the "Lengthen and Release" section on page 162.

All the exercises begin in sitting, standing, supine, prone, kneeling or side-lying positions. Familiarize yourself with the alignment of each position before attempting the exercises. Notice the various cues and images we have given to help you rebalance and develop your body awareness. And always remember to warm up before you start.

Reconnect with your body daily

SITTING ON
A CHAIR >>

Exercises in the sitting position are easy to integrate into your day if you spend a lot of time sitting.

>> Keep your knees in line with your hips and feet flat on the floor, toes pointing forward. Make sure your second toe is pointing straight ahead.

>> Feel the three points of each foot (the bottom of your big toe, the little toe joint and the center of the heel bone) melting evenly into the floor and keep the knees pointing straight over the second toe.

>> Feel your sit bones dropping directly into the chair, not forward or behind you.

>> Find a sense of length in the lower back (lumbar) and float the crown of the head upward to create a space between the ears and shoulders (this should make your body's height increase).

>> Rest your hands on your thighs or place your fingers on the top of your head, palms facing down, with elbows pointing sideways.

>> Align your ears over your sit bones.

>> The back should be broad and wide, with the tips of your shoulder blades broadening sideways and your collarbones opening.

>> In this position you can work on spinal, pelvic and upper body exercises before introducing weight bearing and leg alignment.

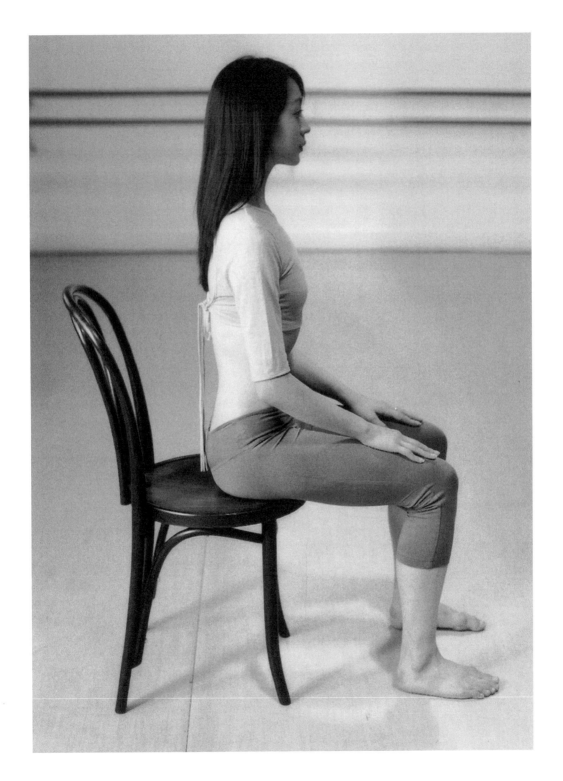

SITTING

CROSS-LEGGED >>

>> Feel your sit bones dropping
into the floor like the roots of
a tree and lengthen the neutral
spine upward along the vertical
alignment through the crown of
your head. Find a sense of length
in the lower back.

>> Rest the hands on the knees,
with your shoulder tips and
collarbones broadening sideways.

ATTENTION TO DETAIL *Keep the
pelvic bowl balanced (see page 11).*

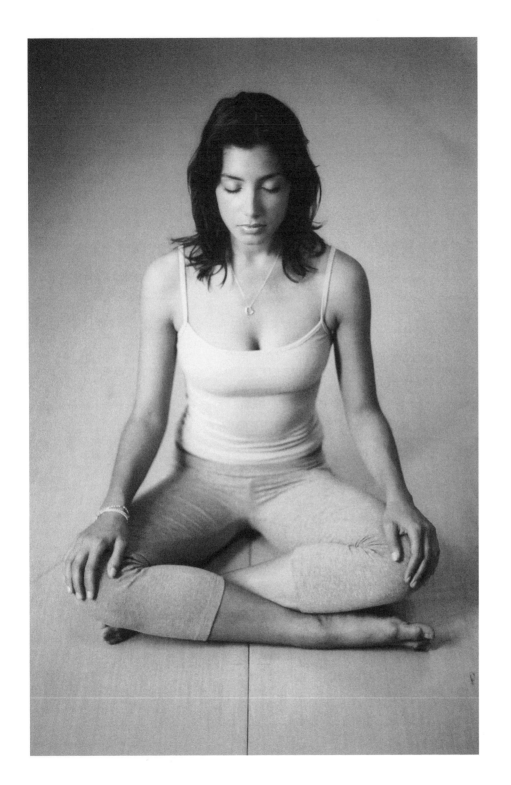

SUPINE >>

>> Lie on your back, knees bent and feet flat.

>> Become aware of the back of the skull and ribs resting on the floor.

>> Notice how your breath affects the contact of the ribs on the floor; the last two ribs may be slightly off the floor at times.

>> Let your pelvis feel heavy and rest your tailbone gently on the floor.

>> Direct your sit bones toward the heels. Make sure they are not pointing to the ceiling or floor.

>> Make sure your hip bones are level on a horizontal line, not lifted or twisted

>> Apply even pressure into the floor through the three points of each foot, with the toes pointing directly forward.

>> Point the knees to the ceiling and keep them in line with your second toe.

>> There should be no surface muscular tension. Imagine the bones melting into the floor.

>> The arms can either be bent at a 90-degree angle with the elbows in line with the shoulders, as shown in the photograph, or placed by your sides with palms facing either the ceiling or the floor.

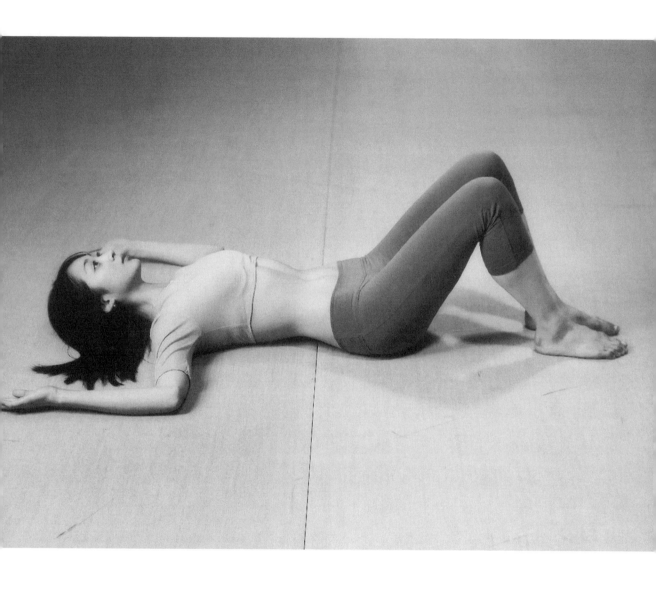

STANDING ⟫

⟫ Direct your sit bones over the heels, pointing them directly toward the floor. Keep the pelvic bowl balanced.

⟫ Feel the weight of the body evenly distributed through the three points of the foot with your center of gravity falling through the front of each ankle.

⟫ Lengthen through the front and back of the legs by visualizing the distance between the heels and sit bones increasing. Don't "lock" the legs straight. Keep the knees soft so they can absorb differences in leg lengths and hip and spinal imbalances. This will also help bring bowlegs and swayback legs into better alignment.

⟫ Try to keep the knees pointing over the second toes as much as possible. The hip bones should be level on the horizontal alignment, not lifted or twisted.

⟫ Align the ears over your sit bones. Don't worry if it feels as though your weight is slightly forward. Remember, we generally move by going forward, so this alignment is a "ready to move" alignment. This is efficient and helps the deep unit do its job.

⟫ Let go of any muscular surface tension and become aware of a sense of "balanced" work all over.

⟫ Try to relax and visualize the muscles falling from the bones to the floor.

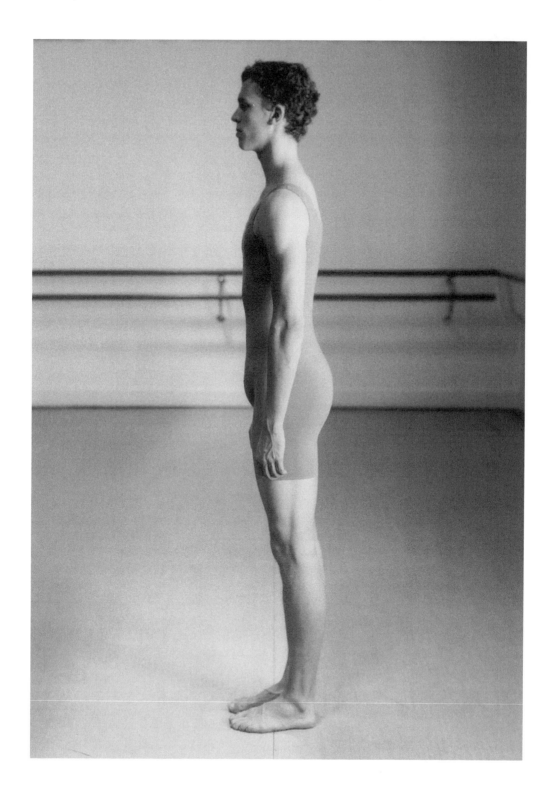

PRONE >>

>> Lie facedown on the floor.

>> Rest your forehead on your fingernails, elbows pointing sideways. This makes a diamond shape and gives the upper chest a gentle opening. Relax the chest into the floor. Alternatively the arms can lie in a wide V shape with the palms and forehead resting on the floor.

>> Relax and allow all the bones to fall through the floor. Don't push or press.

>> You should feel the pubic bone on the floor and be aware of both hip bones being level on a horizontal line.

>> Allow the spine to rest, respecting the natural curves of your spine.

>> The legs can either be together or at a comfortable distance apart, creating a V shape. With the legs together the heel bones can fall away from each other toward the floor. When the legs are apart in a V shape the heels can fall toward each other to the floor. This is a relaxing posture from which to move and should have as little surface tension as possible. Remember to breathe. Just lying in this posture can help you if you habitually sit or hunch over in your daily life.

>> You can place small folded hand towel under your chest if the tightness there is uncomfortable. Over time you can remove or unfold the towel as the chest opens.

>> Remember to be patient and to work slowly toward your goals. Observation is your best tool.

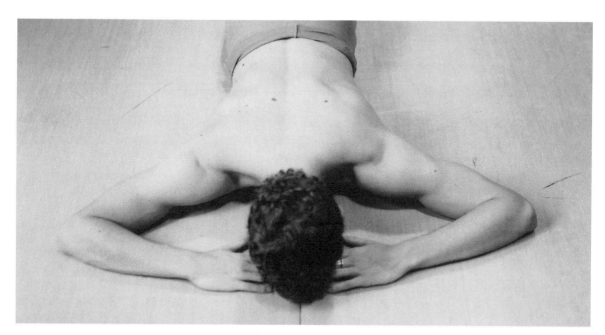

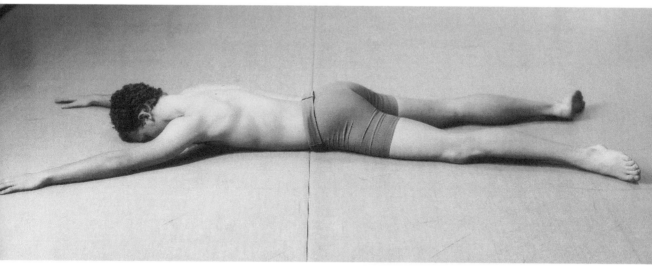

FOUR-POINT
KNEELING »

Four-point kneeling is one of
the more difficult positions to
grasp. Check your alignment
in a mirror.

» Place the hands under the
shoulders and the knees under
the hips with the legs in parallel
alignment.

» Distribute the weight of your body
evenly over the four points of the
hands and knees.

» Keep the spine long and neutral,
taking care to respect the natural
curves. Feel length along the
vertical line through the crown of
the head and tailbone.

» Keep the neck long and maintain
a distance between the ears and
shoulders.

» Be careful not to hyperextend
the elbows.

» Keep the upper back between
the shoulder blades broad and
widening.

» Point your sit bones directly
behind you, not to the floor
or ceiling.

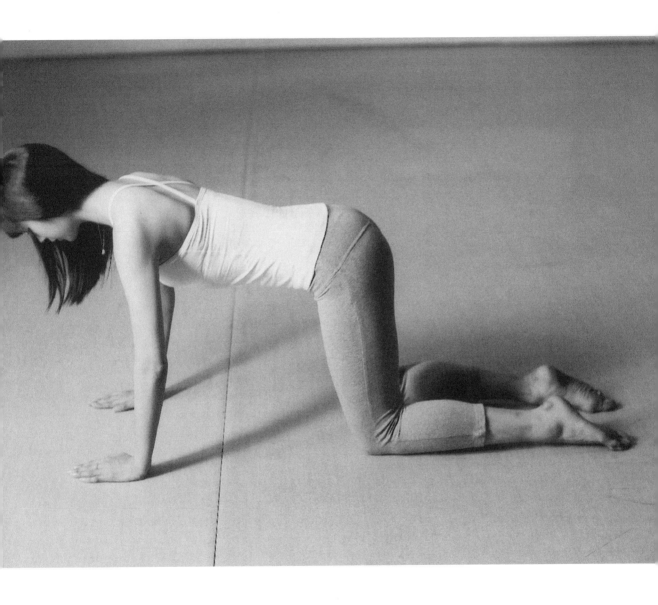

SIDE-LYING >>

>> Lie on your side, knees slightly bent, underneath arm outstretched, with the back of the skull, sit bones and heels aligned along one line.

>> Lay the head gently on the underneath arm and place the other hand on the floor in front of the breastbone or on the top hip.

>> Keep the spine long and neutral.

>> Gently lift the waist from the floor to keep the hips level and horizontal.

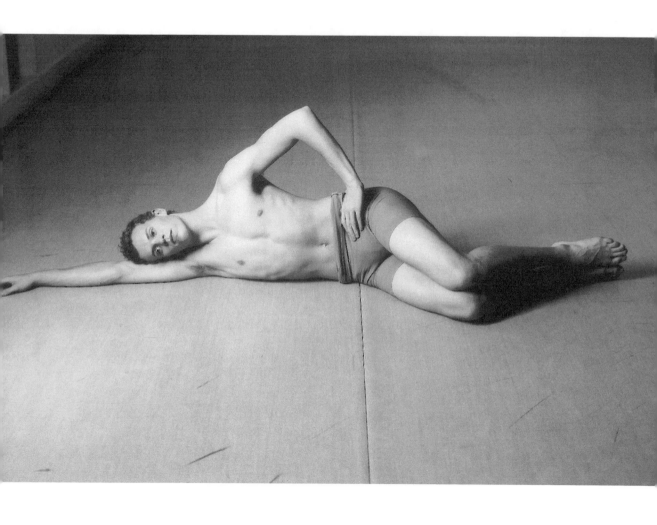

>>awakening

breathing

spinal waves

deep unit work

the body

>> Observational exercises

>> Observing the effect on your collarbones
Align your bones in the sitting position.
Place your hands on your collarbones.
Observe and listen to your breath.
Notice whether your collarbones rise and fall as you breathe.

Use these
exercises to
observe what
happens naturally
in your body
when you breathe.
There is no right
or wrong here—
let the breath
move you!

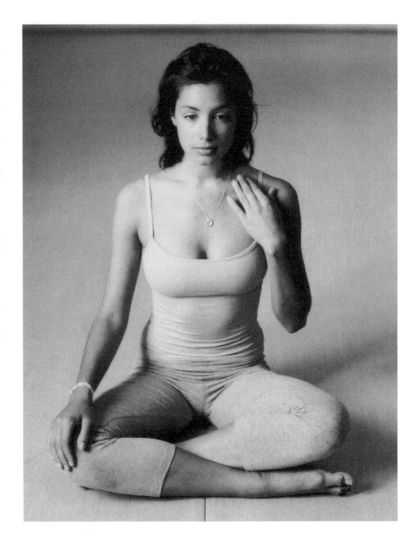

>> Observing effect on the sides of your ribs

Align your bones in the sitting position.
Place hands gently on the sides of your ribs,
with fingers pointing toward the front, thumbs
pointing back, elbows to the side and palms
facing the floor.
Observe and listen to your breath.
Notice the movement of your ribs.

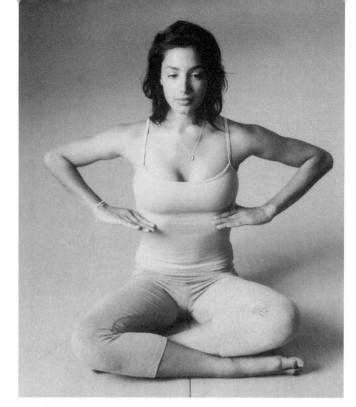

>> Observing the effect on your stomach

Align your bones in the sitting position.
Place the palms of your hands gently
on your stomach.
Observe and listen to your breath.
Notice the movement of your stomach.

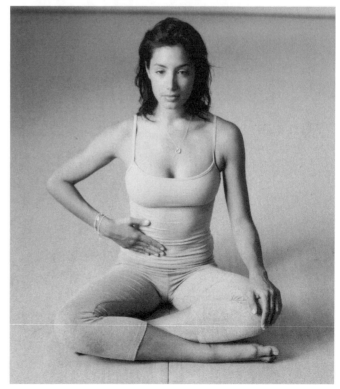

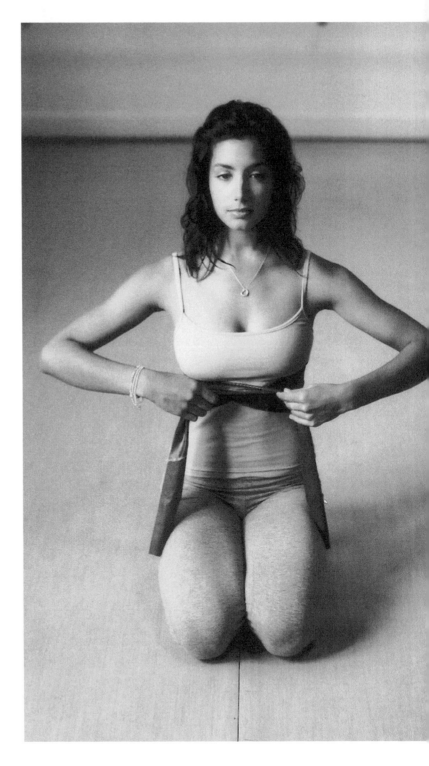

>> Observing the effect on the back of your ribs using an elastic exercise band

Align your bones in the sitting position.

Place an elastic exercise band across the back of your ribs and bring to the front, slightly overlapping against the ribs at the front. Observe and listen to your breath.

ATTENTION TO DETAIL *Notice whether your back expands or whether your hands move away and toward each other.*

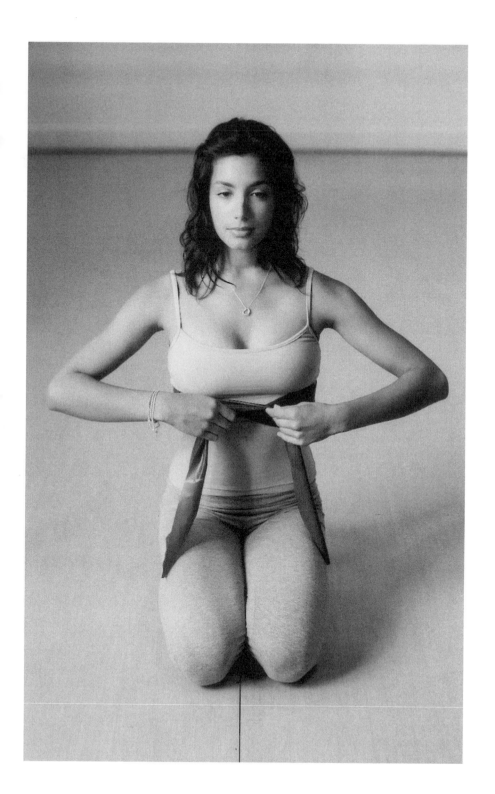

>> Observing the effect on the back of your ribs with a partner

Place your hands on the back of a partner's ribs just below the shoulder blades.
Observe the movement.
Change places.

>> Breathing sideways into the ribs with awareness

Because dancers try to dance with a sense of broadness across their back and they try to make their movements seem effortless, they develop the technique of breathing into the sides and back of their ribs. Now that you have observed the effect your breath can have on different parts of the upper body, try breathing laterally into the ribs. This will encourage a fuller breath.

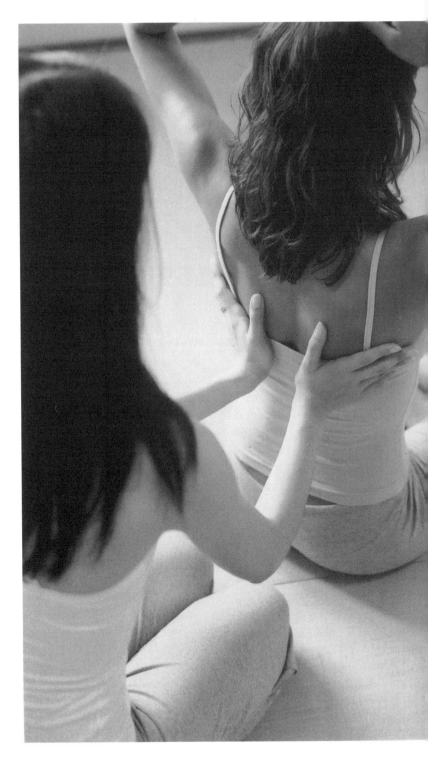

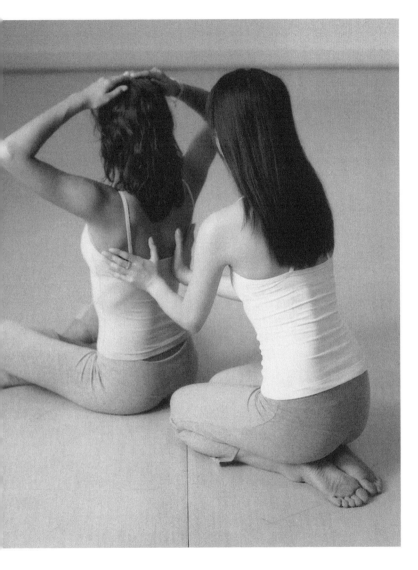

Align your bones in the sitting position.
Place hands gently on the sides of your ribs, with fingers pointing front, thumbs pointing back, elbows to the side and palms facing the floor. While maintaining contact between hands and ribs, actively try to expand the ribs sideways into the hands.

ATTENTION TO DETAIL *Be careful not to "overbreathe." Keep the breath natural. If you experience any shortness of breath or suffer from asthma or breathing disorders, please seek medical advice.*

Awareness test

While maintaining the sideways breath, place your hands on your collarbones and then on your stomach to see if you notice a decrease in the movement in these areas compared to the first time you practiced it. The sideways breath should feel full and give the feeling of broadness across the back.

SPINAL WAVE IN
SUPINE POSITION >>

The following spinal wave exercises are designed to help you discover your neutral spinal alignment and observe and explore your postural boundaries.

Though you may have very little movement to begin with, these movements should feel loose and free.

>> Align your bones in the supine position, with your arms bent at a 90-degree angle, elbows in line with shoulders. Remember to direct your sit bones and toes to the wall in front of your feet.

>> Begin to move the pelvis by directing your sit bones toward the ceiling. You will feel the middle of your back press into the floor.

>> Move in the opposite direction, sending your sit bones down to the floor. You will feel the middle of you back come away from the floor. You have now completed one *spinal wave*.

>> Repeat the spinal waves until you become aware of the reflected movement through your spine. Notice which bones leave and contact the floor. Notice when you feel lengthened and shortened.

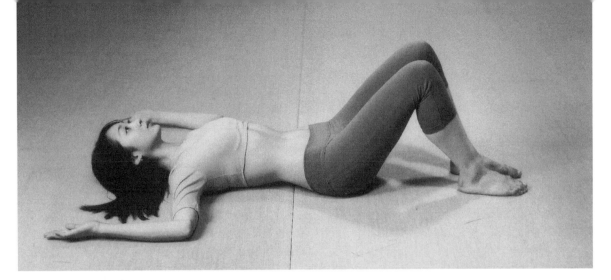

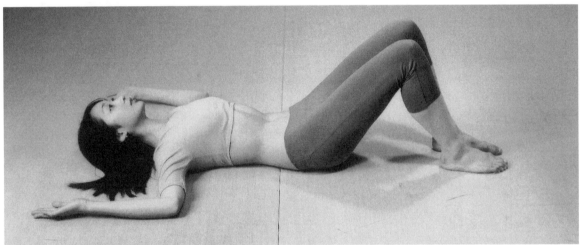

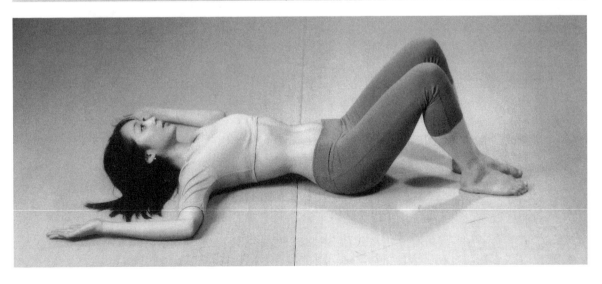

SPINAL WAVE
SITTING ON
CHAIR OR BALL »

>> Align your bones in the sitting position, with your hands resting on thighs or placed on hips, and use your fingers to monitor activity in the oblique muscles. Remember to drop your sit bones toward the floor and lengthen the natural curves of the spine.

>> Begin to move the pelvis by directing your sit bones forward to the wall in front of you.

>> Now move in the opposite direction sending your sit bones behind you.

>> You have now completed one *spinal wave*.

>> Repeat the spinal waves until you become aware of how your height is affected by the position of your pelvis and the reflected movement through your spine. Notice when you feel lengthened and shortened.

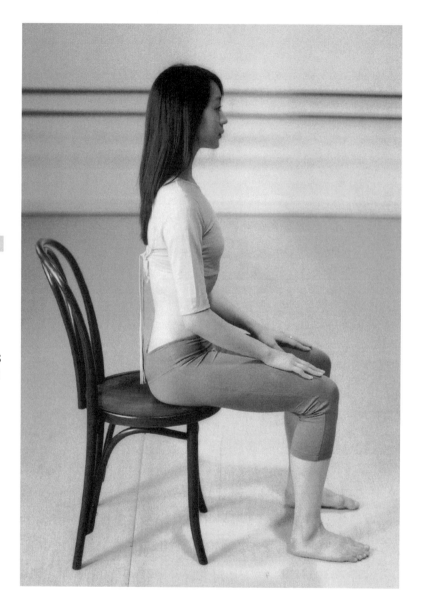

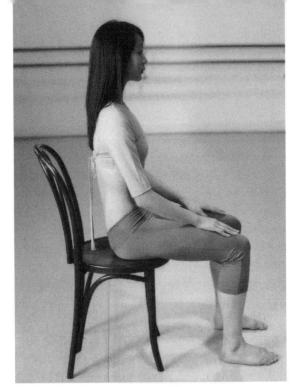

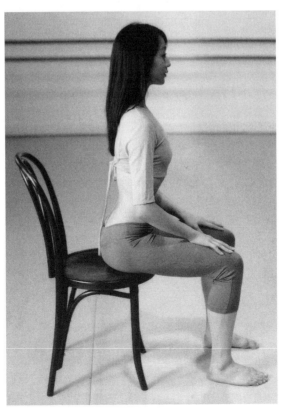

SPINAL WAVE
IN STANDING
POSITION >>

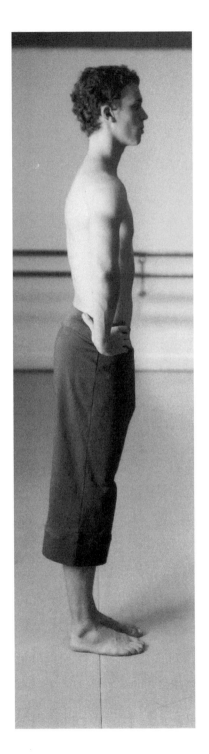

>> Align your bones in the standing position, with hands on hips and use your fingers to monitor activity in the oblique muscles. Remember to direct your sit bones toward the floor, lengthen the natural curves of the spine and soften the knees.

>> Begin to move the pelvis by directing your sit bones forward to the wall in front of you.

>> Now move in the opposite direction, sending your sit bones toward the wall behind you.

>> You have now completed one *spinal wave.*

>> Repeat the spinal waves until you become aware of how your height is affected by the position of your pelvis and the reflected movement through your spine and knees. Notice when you feel lengthened and shortened.

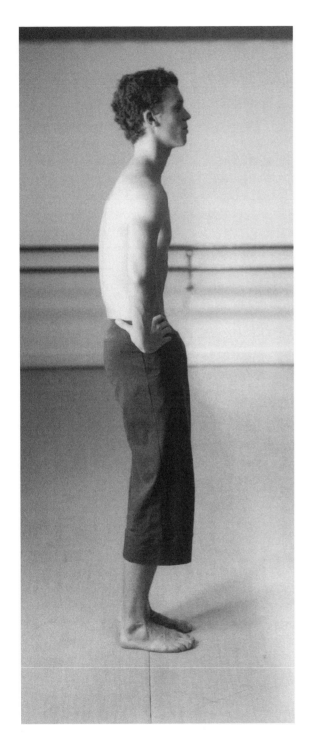
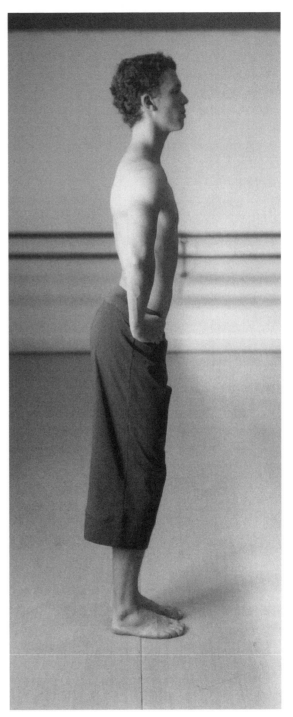

DIAMOND-SHAPED PULL-UPS FOR PELVIC FLOOR AWARENESS >>

>> Sit cross-legged on the floor and align your bones in the sitting position.

>> Visualize the diamond shape of the pelvic floor muscles, as outlined on page 15.

>> Gently draw the center of the diamond upward.

>> Hold this lift and breathe naturally for up to ten breaths.

>> Release the muscle and begin again.

>> If you lose the feeling of the upward pull before ten breaths, simply relax and start again.

>> You can practice these pulls as often as you like in sitting and standing postures.

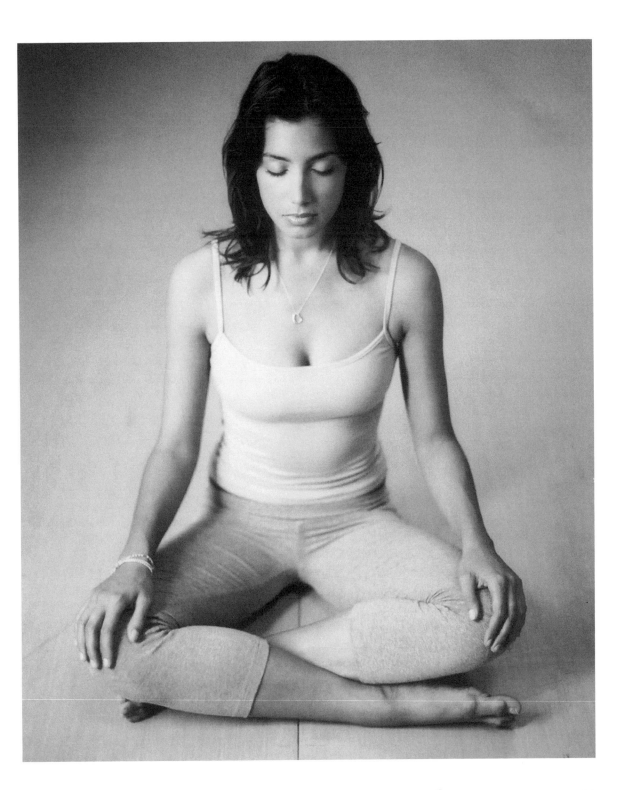

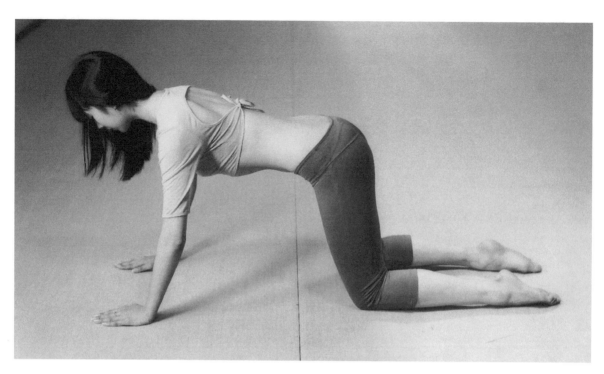

DEEP AND GENTLE
ABDOMINAL
LIFTS 》

This is a gentle exercise to activate the TA.

》 Align your bones in the four-point kneeling position. Maintain length along the natural curves of the spine and keep your sit bones pointing directly behind you.

》 As you breathe in allow the belly to relax and hang toward the floor.

》 As you breathe out bring the belly button gently up toward the spine and multifidus.

》 Try to maintain the belly button toward the spine while taking several natural breaths.

》 Repeat this up to ten times.

ATTENTION TO DETAIL *Be careful not to let the spine arch when you release the belly and watch that you don't overactivate the obliques when you take the belly button to the spine.*

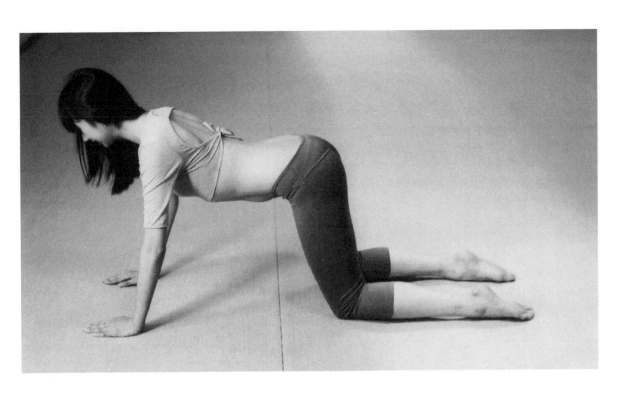

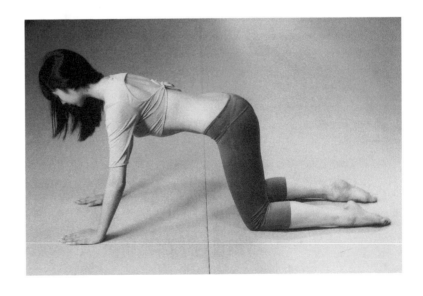

>>mobilizing

the body

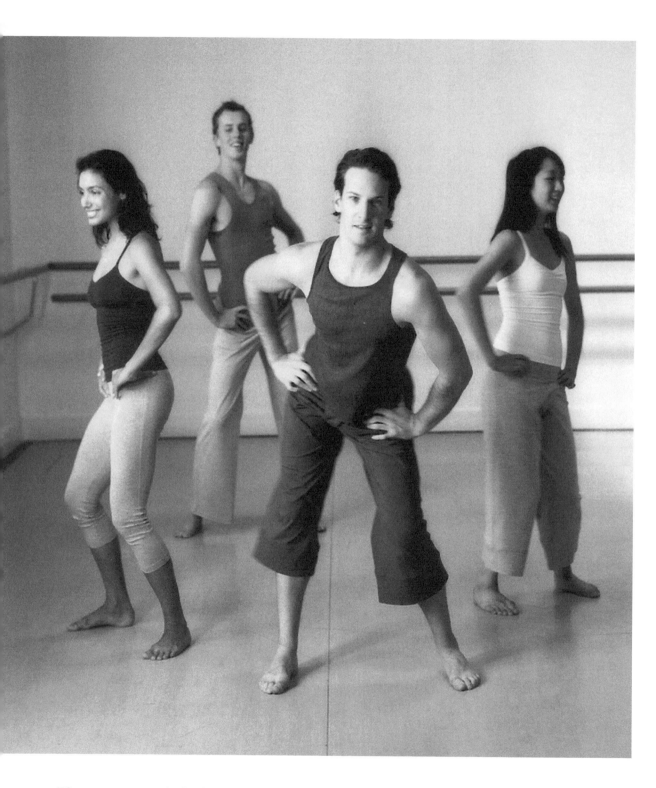

« ballet-fit workout »

FIGURE EIGHTS
FOR HIPS »

This is a good gentle mobilizer of the hips, lower back, pelvis and knees. It eases overtense hips and releases the rectus femoris (the muscle that runs from the pelvis to the knee).

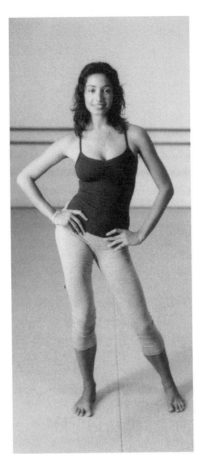
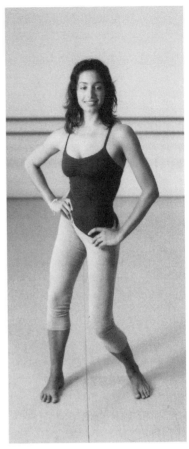

>> Align your bones in the standing position with your feet slightly wider than your hips. Place your hands on your hips and slightly bend the knees.

>> Imagine your sit bones are beams of light pointing toward the floor. Draw imaginary figure eights on the floor with the beams of light. Start your figure eights forward to the left or right and change the way you start each session. Draw your figure eights sideways on the floor horizontally as well as vertically.

>> Gradually move the figure eights so that the sit bones are pointing to the wall behind you. Lean forward to counterbalance your weight.

>> Gradually return, bringing your sit bones back to pointing toward the floor.

>> Draw ten figure eights clockwise and ten counterclockwise.

>> Increase the size of the figure eights as you become more comfortable with this exercise.

FOLDING IN
FRONT OF HIP >>

This exercise can be very beneficial if you stand or are on your feet a great deal.

>> Align your bones in the standing position, with your hands on your hips.

>> Bend the knees and move the heels sideways to inwardly rotate the legs and feet.

>> Let your sit bones swing back toward the wall behind you, making a deep fold at the front of the hips.

>> Lean forward to counterbalance your weight.

>> Let the legs inwardly rotate, with the knees falling toward each other.

>> You can move in and out of the fold up to ten times or rest into it for several breaths.

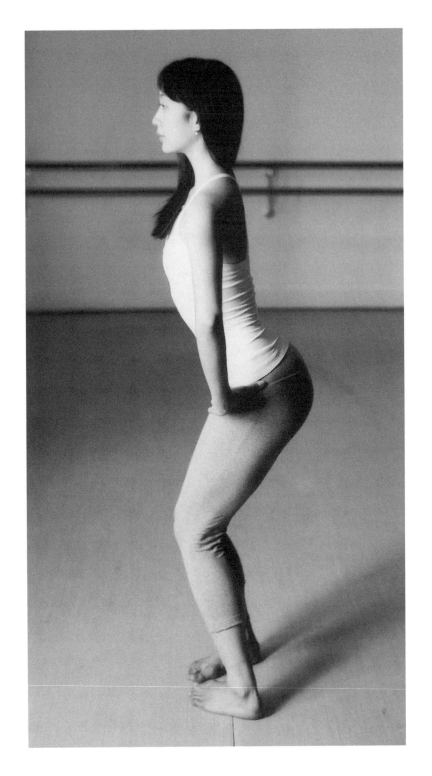

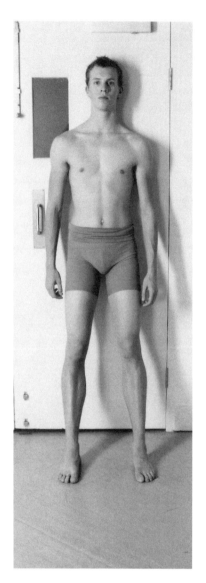
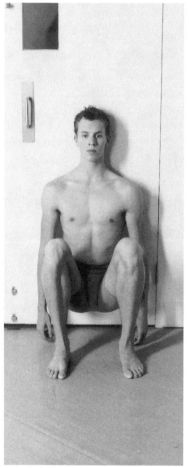
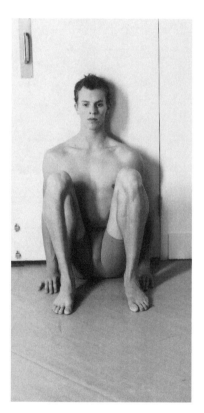

« ballet-fit workout »

WALL SLIDE >>

This exercise releases
hip tension.

>> Stand with your back against
a wall, feet slightly away from
it and hip-width apart.

>> Bend your knees and slide your
back down the wall, maintaining
a neutral spinal alignment. Feel
the back of your head, ribs and
tailbone against the wall for
as long as possible. Keep your
sit bones dropping directly to
the floor.

>> As you slide your sit bones
toward the floor, relax the front of
the hips to create a deep
fold and crease.

>> Slide down as far as you can
without moving your feet. Once
your buttocks touch the ground,
extend your legs out in front of
you so that you are sitting
comfortably on the floor. If your
buttocks do not touch the
ground, simply walk one foot
forward at a time until you are
sitting. Bend your knees and roll
onto your hands and knees.
Move your weight backward onto
your feet in order to begin rolling
up through the spine to standing.

>>Repeat this up to five times.

FIGURE EIGHT
ARM SWINGS »

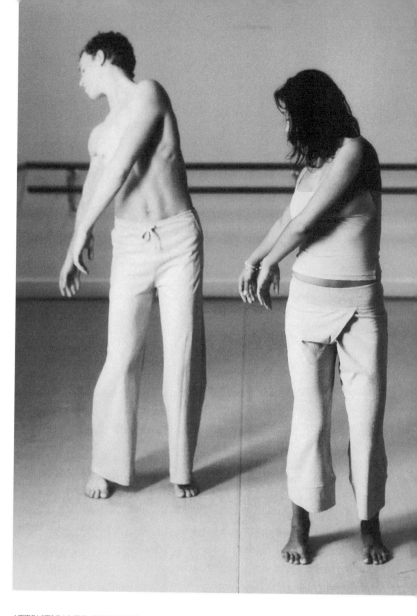

This exercise gently releases
and mobilizes the spine.

» Align your bones in the
standing position.

» Soften the knees and swing the
arms diagonally across the body,
with fingers dropping toward
the floor.

» Lift your arms up to the ceiling,
extending the legs, and begin to
turn your head to the other side.

» Soften the knees and swing
the arms diagonally down across
the body to begin making figure
eight patterns in the air on the
other side.

ATTENTION TO DETAIL *Keep
movements loose and relaxed and feel
the weight of the bones as they fall and
swing. Experiment with your natural
breath to assist in finding a rhythm for
this exercise.*

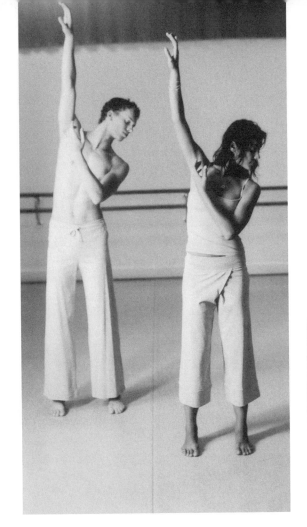

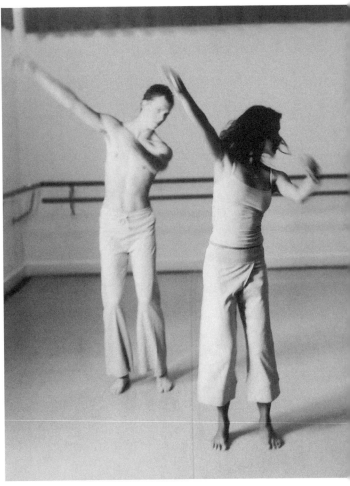

>> efficient

abdominals

KNEE FALLS TO THE SIDE >>

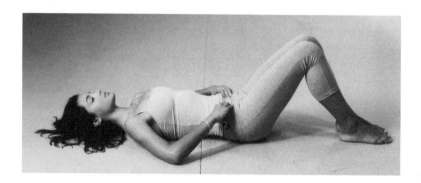

This exercise works your deepest stabilizers, so stay relaxed and give these deep muscles a workout. Keep the focus on your bones.

Remember to monitor the activity of your superficial abdominal muscles.

>> Align your bones in the supine position, with your hands on your hips, and use your fingers to monitor the activity in the oblique muscles.

>> Let your knee fall gently to the side without activating the oblique muscles and without moving the pelvic bones. As the leg falls sideways feel the weight of the thighbone falling into the hip socket and don't allow any movement of the other leg. If the obliques switch on, modify the range of the falling knee. Only move the knee as far as it will go comfortably. The range will increase with practice.

>> Return the working leg to its original position.

>> Do this ten times with the first leg, then repeat with the other.

ATTENTION TO DETAIL *Be careful not to hold your breath. Breathe naturally.*

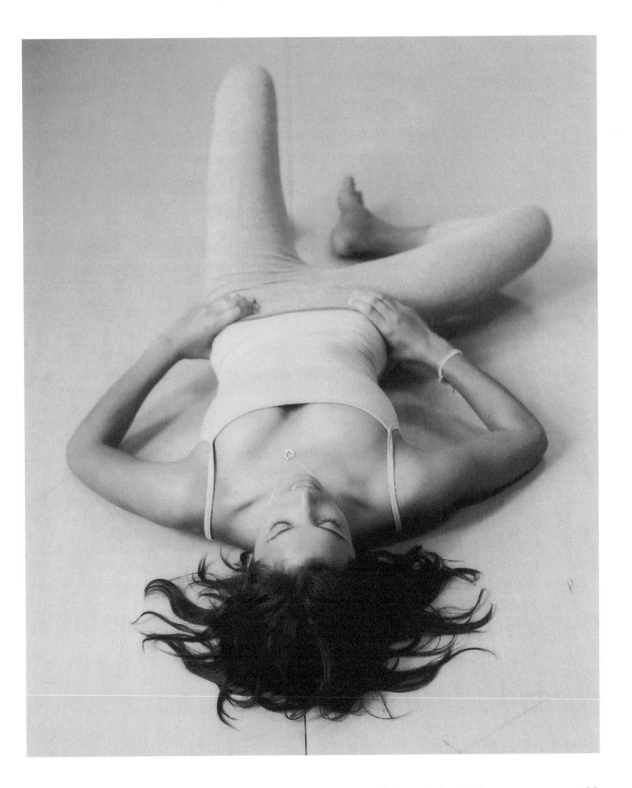

LEG SLIDES
AND FLOATS »

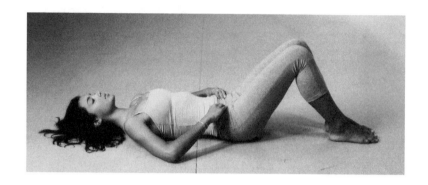

This exercise is used as a deep unit awakener. Monitor the activity in your obliques, keeping them as soft as possible (see page 15). Your ability to do this will improve with practice.

» Align your bones in the supine position, with your hands on your hips, and use your fingers to monitor activity in the oblique muscles.

» Slowly extend the leg by sliding it along the floor in front of you, reaching the sides of the heel bone away from your sit bones.

» Gently press the heel bone of the extended leg into the floor to activate the hamstring and then reverse the leg slide until the foot floats up from the floor.

» Keep bending the knee until you feel the leg bone drop into the hip socket, creating a deep fold in the front of the hip. You have now completed one leg float.

» Slide the leg along the floor again to begin the next float.

» Repeat ten times with the first leg and then the other.

» Try using one breath for the extension and one for the knee bend and then reverse the breath.

ATTENTION TO DETAIL *Make sure there is no tension on the outside of the thigh or around the hip. Keep the obliques soft throughout because this will encourage the deeper iliopsoas muscle to do the work.*

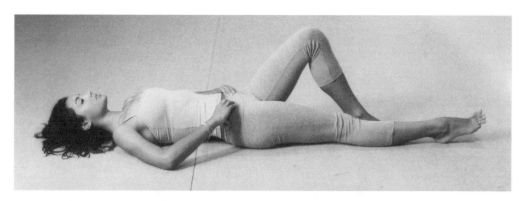

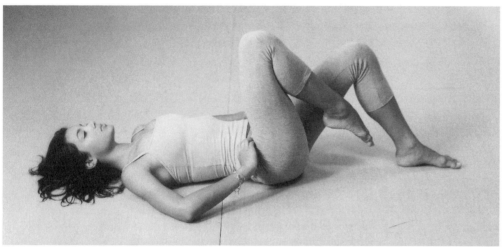

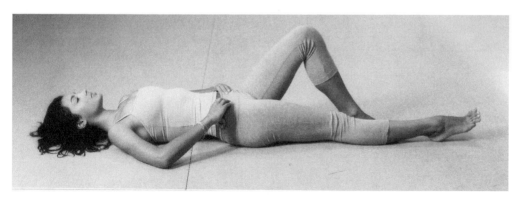

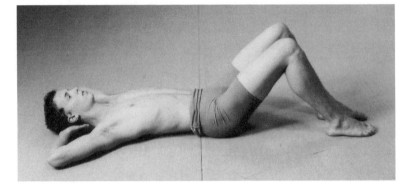

CURL-UPS WITH
OBLIQUE TWISTS »

This exercise is designed to explore the range of movement of the obliques. Try coordinating one breath for each movement. Encourage the abdominal muscles to relax at the beginning and end of each movement.

» Align your bones in the supine position, with the tips of the fingers meeting at the back of the head. Elbows out to the side in line with the ears.

» Softly take your chin toward your chest and begin to curl the upper spine until the tips of the shoulder blades are just touching the floor.

» Begin to twist to the right, taking the left elbow directly to the ceiling and the right elbow just off the floor, diagonally away from the right shoulder.

» Reverse the movement back to the floor.

» Repeat to the other side and continue alternating up to five times on each side.

ATTENTION TO DETAIL *The pelvis and knees should remain still throughout this exercise. Stop if you experience neck pain. Make sure you do not lift the shoulders during the curl up. Do not pull the head forward. Keep the hands flat.*

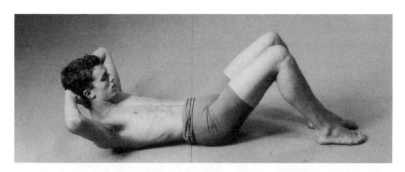

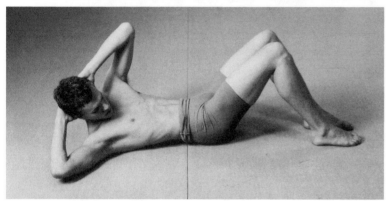

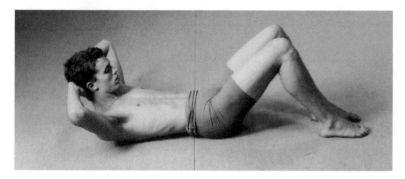

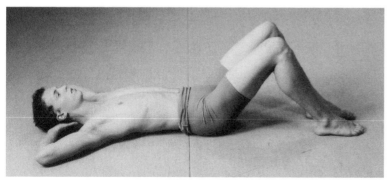

SCISSOR LEGS >>

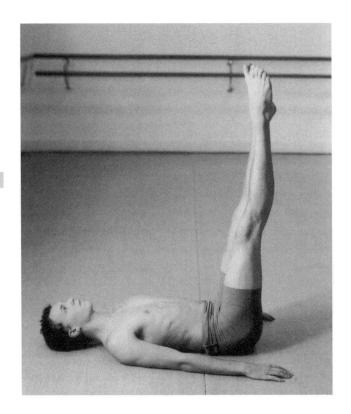

You can increase the range and speed of your legs when you feel confident with maintaining neutral spinal alignment. Scissor legs can also be done without the curl up if your abdominal muscles are not yet strong. When you feel confident, this exercise can also be used as an effective warm-up.

>> Align your bones in the supine position.

>> Extend the legs, one at a time, up to the ceiling, making a 90-degree angle to the body.

>> Stretch the knees as much as possible, reach the toes to the ceiling and rotate the legs gently outward.

>> Softly take your chin toward your chest and begin to curl the upper spine until the tips of the shoulder blades are just touching the ground, with your hands reaching up toward the knees.

>> Move the legs in a scissorlike motion, forward and back, gently connecting (not holding) the hands to the legs.

>> Maintaining the curl-up, alternate the legs in another scissorlike motion, making sure the heels touch as they pass the midpoint.

>> Continue alternating the legs, maintaining a speed that allows correct execution.

>> Check that you have maintained neutral pelvic alignment, with the sit bones facing the wall, not the ceiling.

ATTENTION TO DETAIL *For this exercise you need to be able to extend the leg from the supine position up to 90 degrees comfortably with no tightness in the back of the leg and without losing the neutral pelvic alignment.*

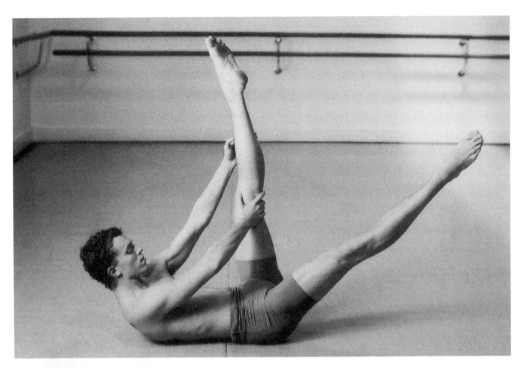

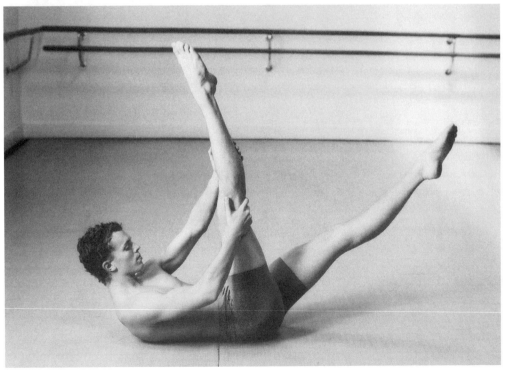

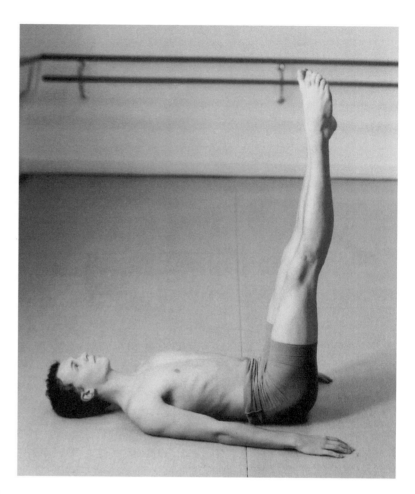

BICYCLE LEGS »

This exercise can also be used in your warm-up session as a mobilizer.

» Align your bones in the supine position.

» Extend the legs, one at a time, up to the ceiling, making a 90-degree angle to the body. The legs should be parallel, with the arms relaxed on the floor.

» Begin to bicycle the legs.

» Maintain neutral spinal alignment, with your sit bones facing the wall, not the ceiling.

» Reach the legs toward the ceiling as you bicycle and keep your movements relaxed. Maintain a consistent speed.

ATTENTION TO DETAIL *Keep the pelvis neutral throughout all the movements.*

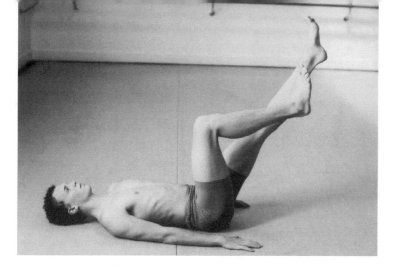

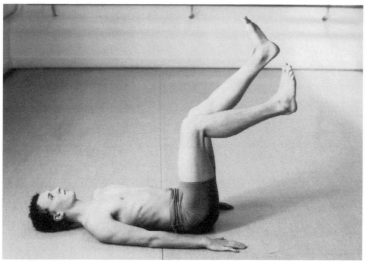

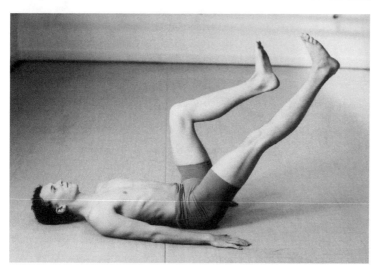

alignm

dynami

robo

>>the articula
exp

aware

holisti

e and
essive back

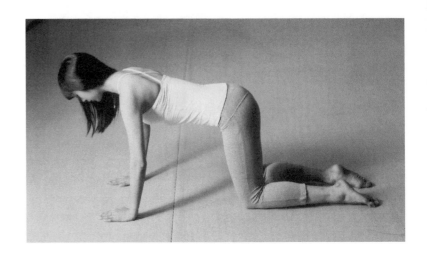

HALF CATS 〉〉

This exercise mobilizes the lower lumbar area of the spine.

〉〉 Align your bones in the four-point kneeling position.

〉〉 Create a small C with your lower back by dropping your tailbone down toward the floor and imagining it gently pulling through your legs, toward your hands.

〉〉 This is a small movement. Don't let it affect your upper back.

〉〉 When you feel the curve move into the lower ribs return to the original position of neutral spinal alignment, finishing with your sit bones pointing toward the wall behind you.

〉〉 Repeat ten times.

ATTENTION TO DETAIL *Be careful not to swing the position forward or hinge back on the arms and legs.*

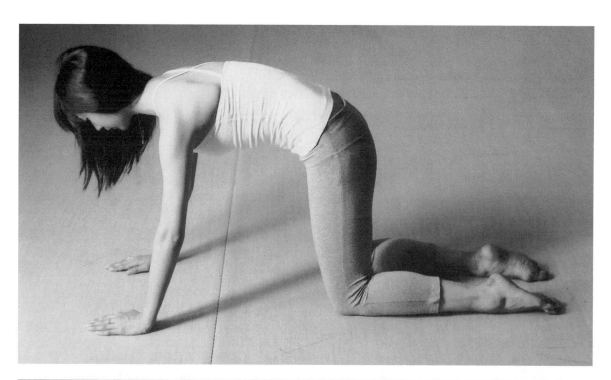

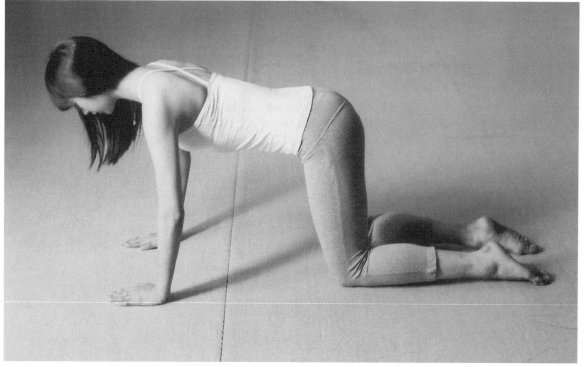

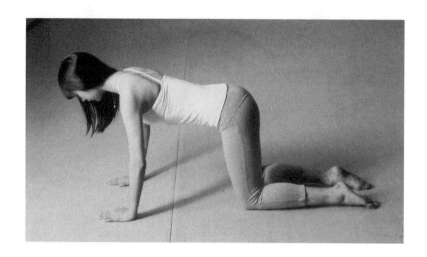

FULL CATS >>

This exercise mobilizes the lower lumbar and upper spine into flexion.

>> Align your bones in the four-point kneeling position.

>> Move into the small C position as for "half cats" (see page 94).

>> Continue the curve into the upper back and allow your head to drop naturally as the entire spine curves.

>> Try to be aware of articulating a single vertebra at a time.

>> Return to the original position of neutral spinal alignment finishing with your sit bones pointing toward the wall behind you.

>> Repeat this ten times.

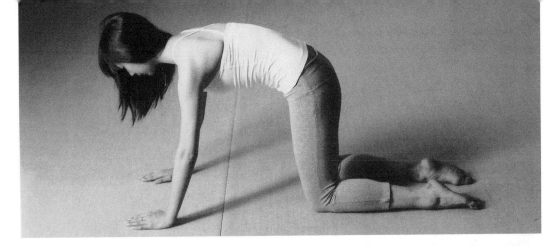

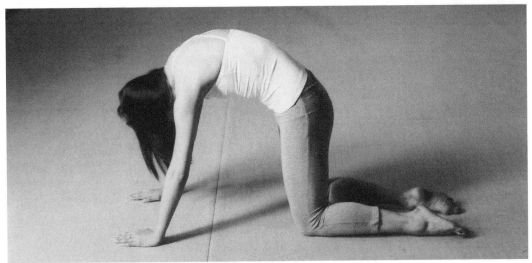

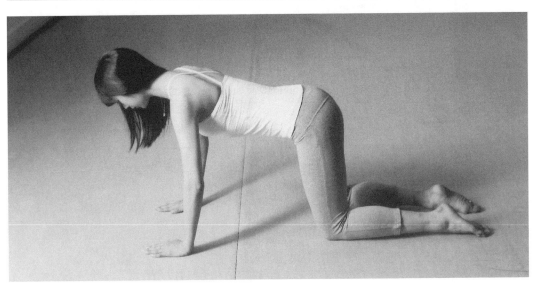

DIAMOND
PRESS >>

This exercise is especially good if you hunch over a desk. It mobilizes and opens the upper back.

>> Align your bones in the prone position, with your forehead resting on your fingernails, palms facing down.

>> Breathe out and relax the whole body into the floor.

>> Begin to gently pull the bottom tips of the shoulder blades down and out toward the armpits.

>> Reach your breastbone along the floor toward the fingertips without lifting off the floor.

>> Try to feel the crown of your head reaching forward.

>> Keep your neck long by not lifting your chin.

>> Continue extending this line of movement by allowing your head to lift slightly away from the fingers.

>> You should feel a broadening across your back and a sense of work between and around the shoulder blades.

>> Maintain this action for one or two natural breaths.

>> Relax and return to the original position.

>> Repeat up to ten times, building your repetitions slowly at first.

ATTENTION TO DETAIL *You should not experience pain in the neck, upper body or lower back. If you have scoliosis or an imbalance in your back muscles you will sense a difference between one side of your back and the other.*

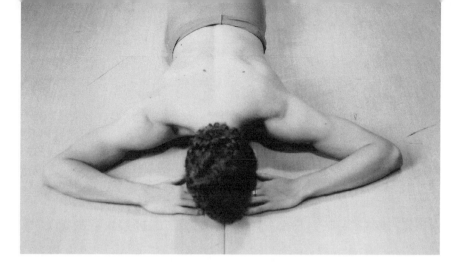

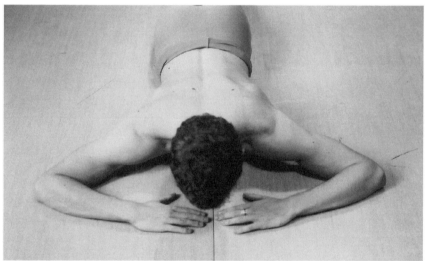

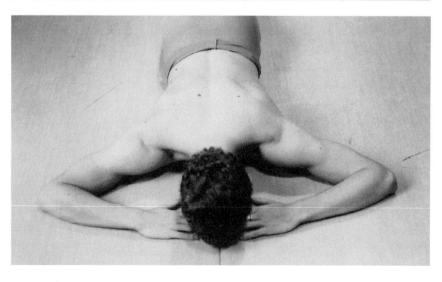

DIAMOND
PRESS, SITTING »

Perform this exercise sideways
to a mirror to check your
alignment.

>> Align your bones in the sitting
position on a chair, with your
hands on your head and elbows
pointing directly to the side.

>> Turn your head to one side.

>> Gently pull the bottom tips of
the shoulder blades down and
out toward the armpits.

>> Reach the breastbone to the
ceiling creating a small arc
through the upper body.

>> Gently pull the tips of the
elbows sideways.

>> Be careful not to lift the chin
out of alignment or arch the
lower back.

>> You should feel a broadening
across your back and a sense
of work between and around
the shoulder blades.

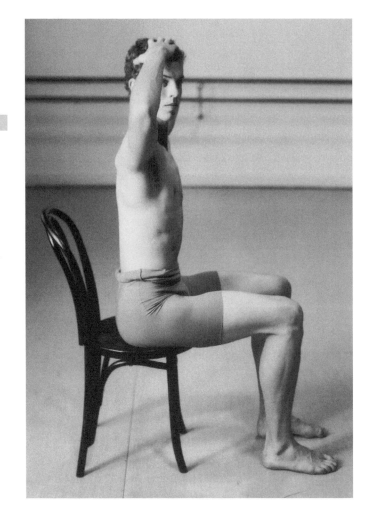

>> Relax and return to the original
position.

>> Repeat up to ten times, turn your
head to the other side and
repeat. Build your repetitions
slowly at first.

ATTENTION TO DETAIL *Make sure
the lower back does not arch and the
lower ribs flare forward. Imagine your
sternum sliding to the ceiling.*

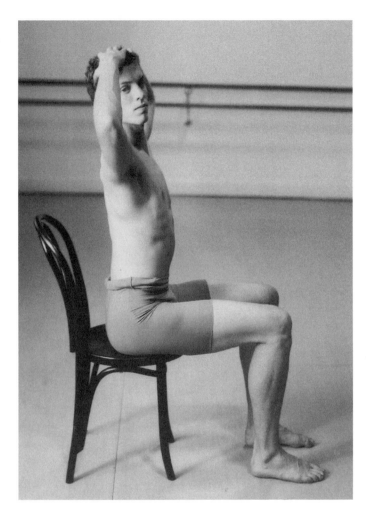

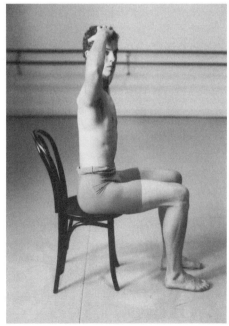

SPINAL ROLL-
DOWN, SITTING »

This exercise is designed
to articulate and create an
awareness of the spine
through flexion.

>> Align your bones sitting on
a chair with hands beside
your knees as shown in
the photograph.

>> Take your chin down toward your
throat and begin to roll down
through the spine allowing the
arms to slide down the sides of
the legs. Articulate the vertebra
as you move through the spine.

>> Keep your sit bones firmly planted
on the chair and only go as far
as you can without letting them
swing backward and come
away from the chair.

>> Reverse the action to return,
initiating the movement by
pulling the belly button in
toward the spine.

>> Repeat up to ten times.

ATTENTION TO DETAIL *Imagine each
vertebra travels up the spine before
spilling up and over toward the floor.*

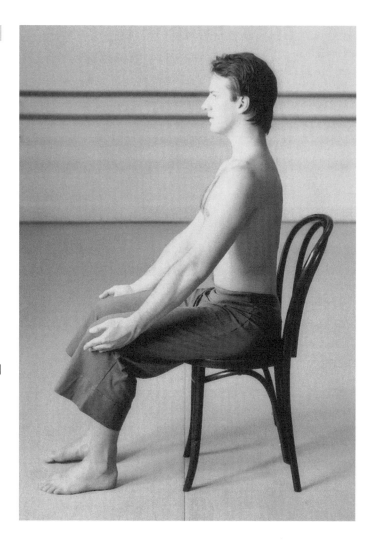

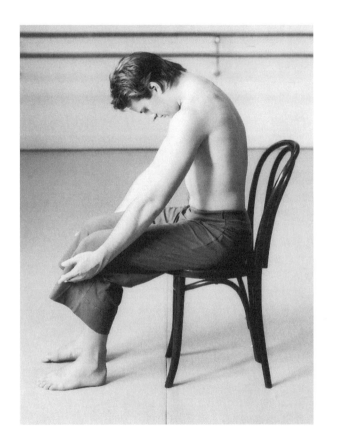
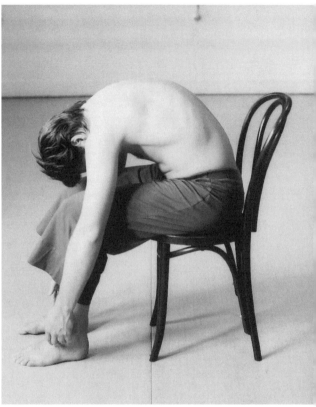

STANDING SPINAL ROLL-DOWN »

This exercise mobilizes the spine and stretches the lower back and the back of the legs. These movements require a large degree of mobility and flexibility of the joints and muscles in the back and legs.

» Align your bones in the standing position.

» Keeping your center of gravity over the front of your ankles, take your chin down toward your throat and begin to roll down through the spine. Keep the crown of your head falling toward the feet and try not to hinge forward at the hips or lower back.

» Articulate each vertebra as you move through the spine until your hands touch the floor.

» Allow the elbows to bend and continue until the crown of your head is as close to the floor as possible. The knees can soften slightly to ease any tightness in the back of the legs.

» Reverse the action to return to the starting position. Initiate the return by pulling the belly button in toward the spine and dropping the tailbone down toward the floor.

» Repeat up to ten times.

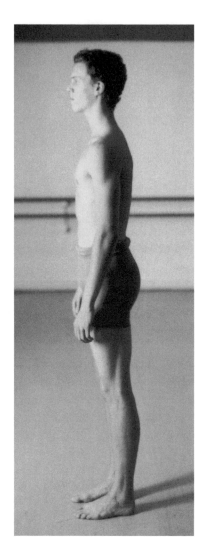

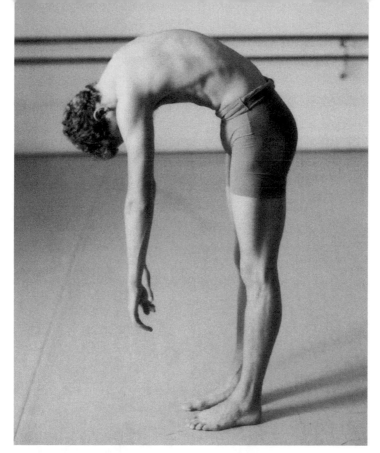

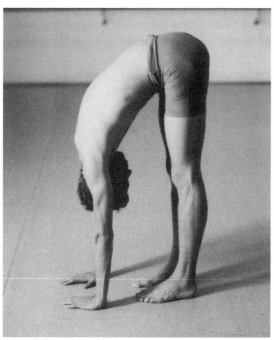

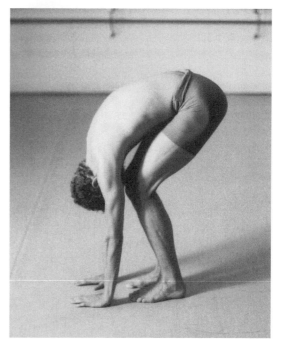

« the articulate and expressive back »   105

SPINAL TWIST »

The following two spinal twist exercises mobilize the spine through rotation.

» Align your bones sitting on a chair with your hands on your head or kneeling as shown in the photograph.

» Imagine your arms radiating sideways from the spine and reach the elbows away from your ears.

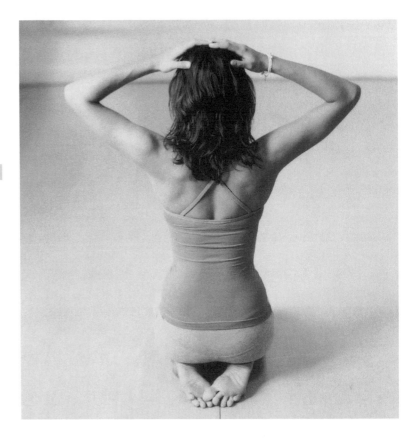

» Keep your sit bones firmly planted on the chair or on your heels if you are kneeling.

» Begin to twist to the right. Move as far as you can, keeping your sit bones dropping downward

» Make sure you spiral on the vertical alignment and keep your hips facing the front.

» Return to the starting position. This is one spinal twist.

» Do this up to ten times, alternating to each side.

ATTENTION TO DETAIL *Keep the movement just rotating. Resist the temptation to side-bend, flex or extend the spine.*

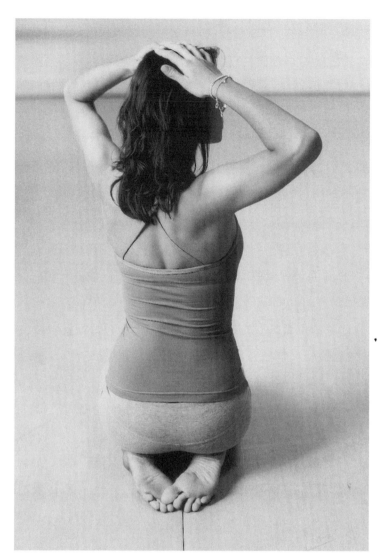

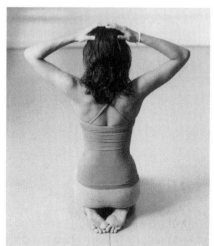

SPINAL TWIST
VARIATION
ON CHAIR >>

>> Sit sideways on a chair with the back of the chair on your right side. Align your bones and sit firmly on the chair with your hands on your head.

>> Begin to twist to the right, as in the "spinal twist" (on page 106).

>> Place your hands on the back of the chair and gently increase the twist. Remember to keep the spine on the vertical alignment.

>> Return to the starting position. This is one spinal twist.

>> Do this no more than five times, alternating each side.

ATTENTION TO DETAIL *To maintain your alignment of the upper body, imagine your elbows are the agitators in a washing machine.*

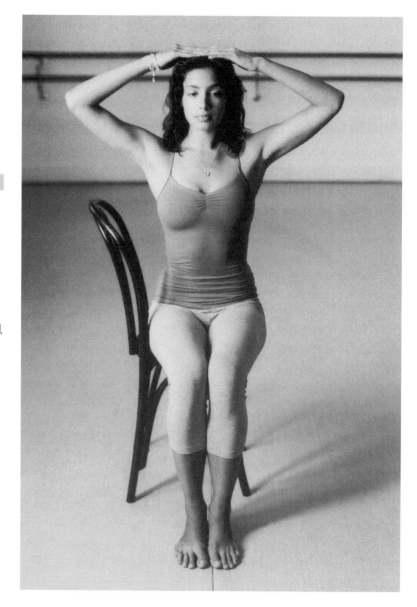

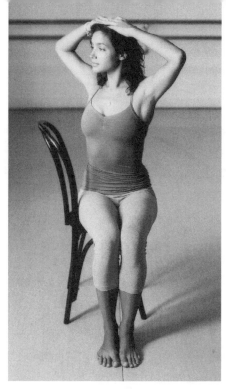
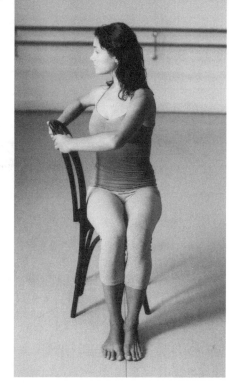
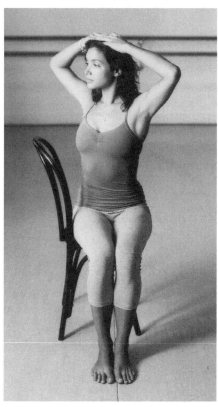
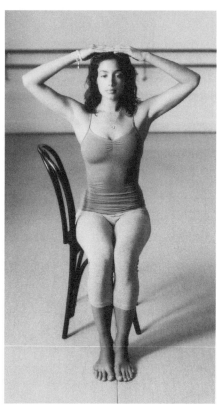

《 the articulate and expressive back 》 109

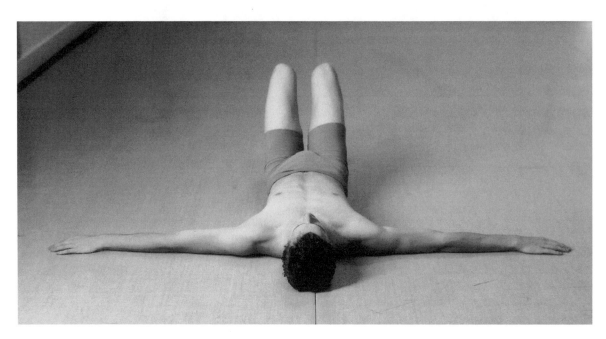

HIP ROLLS FOR
THE SPINE »

This exercise releases tension
and mobilizes the spine.

» Align your bones in the supine
position, with arms outstretched
to the side, palms flat to the floor.
Imagine that between your knees
you are holding a tennis ball that
you must not drop.

» Let your knees fall gently to one
side, toward the floor.

» Let the hips follow your knees,
but keep both shoulder blades
connected to the floor. The head
turns simultaneously in the
opposite direction to the knees.

» Reverse the action back to the
supine position, moving the hips
first, then the knees.

» Repeat this ten times to each
side, alternating sides.

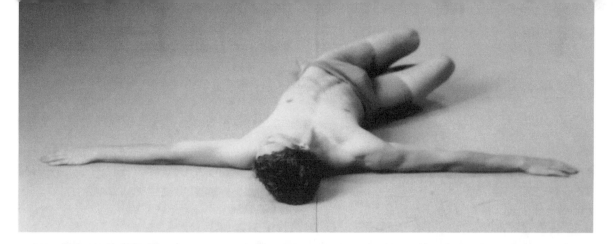

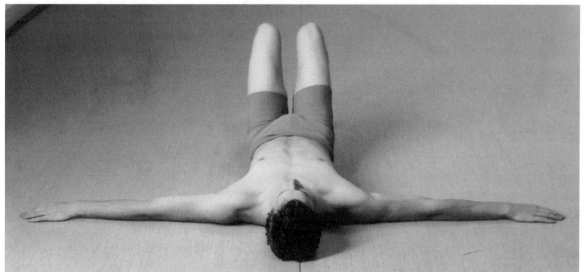

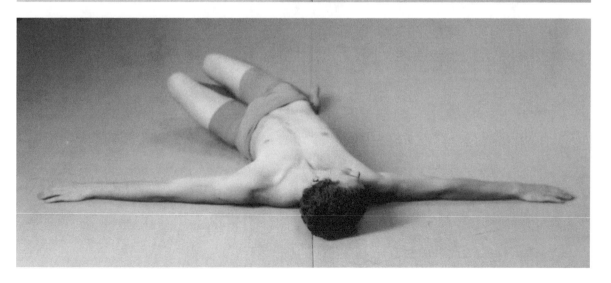

>>from hips

ent
stability
ncing
to toes
balance

KNEE CIRCLES
FOR HIPS >>

This exercise mobilizes the hip joint by working in outward and inward rotation.

>> Align your bones in the supine position with your hands on your hips and use your fingers to monitor activity in the oblique muscles.

>> Float one knee toward the chest to a 90-degree angle without tilting your sit bones toward the ceiling.

>> Feel the weight of the thighbone falling backward into the hip socket.

>> Begin to circle the thighbone at the hip joint either inward or outward by imagining that the kneecap is tracing small circles the size of a nickel on the ceiling.

>> Do ten circles in each direction using one breath for each circle.

>> Repeat to the other side.

ATTENTION TO DETAIL *Keep the oblique muscles soft and be aware of a relaxed feeling in the muscles of the hip.*

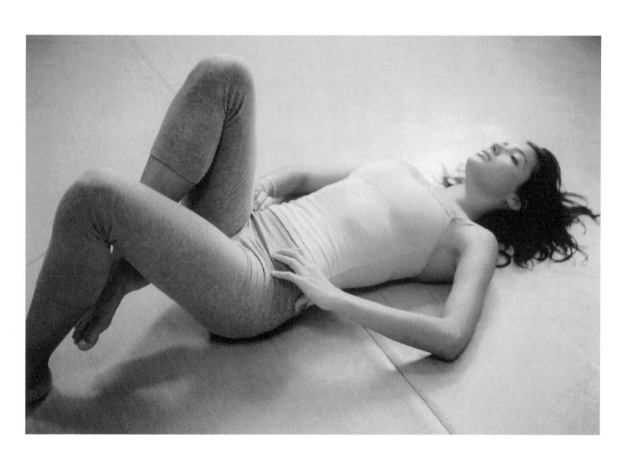

KNEE FALLS TO THE SIDE WITH A FOCUS ON OUTWARD ROTATION ≫

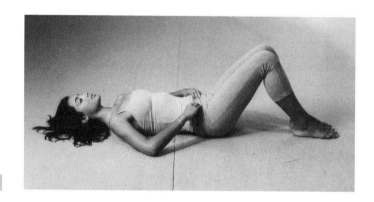

Use this exercise to explore a soft gentle feeling of external rotation in the hip joint.

≫ Align your bones in the supine position with your hands on your hips and use your fingers to monitor activity in the oblique muscles.

≫ Let one knee fall gently to the side without activating the oblique muscles and without moving the pelvic bones. As the leg falls sideways feel the weight of the thighbone falling into the hip socket and don't allow any movement in the other leg.

≫ Focus on the sensation of the leg in outward rotation as it moves in isolation to the pelvis.

≫ Return the leg to its original position.

≫ Do this ten times with the first leg, then repeat with the other leg.

ATTENTION TO DETAIL *Be careful not to hold your breath. Breathe naturally.*

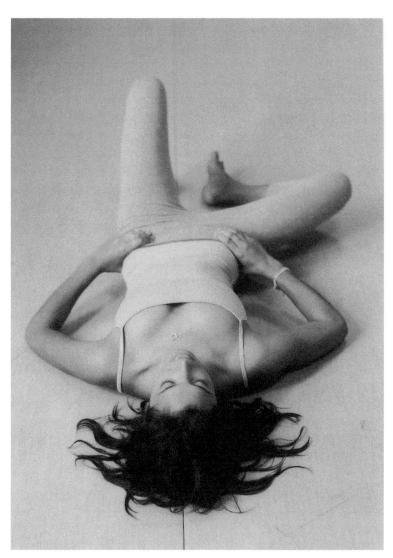

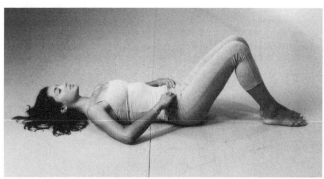

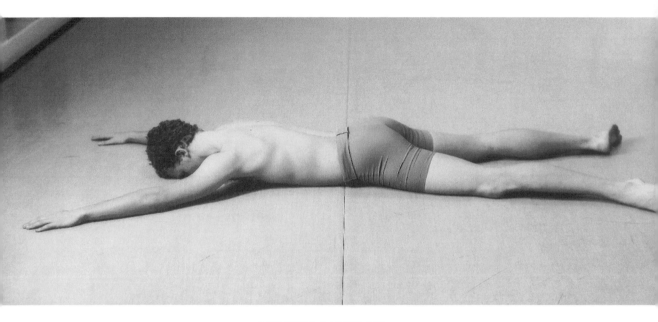

ALTERNATING
LEG REACH »

This exercise is designed to explore the isolation of leg movement in the pelvis.

» Align your bones in the prone position with the arms and legs in a V shape. Legs should be outwardly rotated.

» Begin to pull the inside thigh of the left leg down toward the floor and with a softly stretched foot reach the left heel bone away from the left sit bone.

» Continue these actions until the leg begins to float from the floor. Only reach the leg as far as you can without changing the pelvic alignment. As the leg lifts, maintain the pelvic alignment.

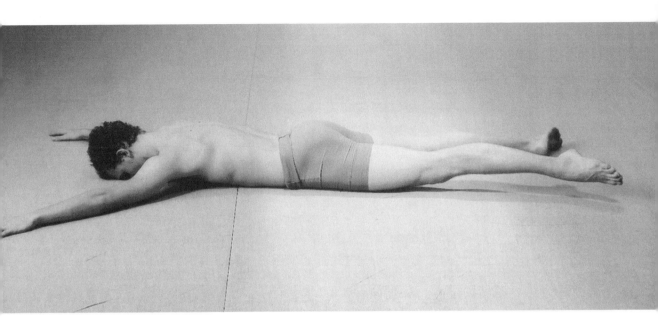

>> Return the leg to the floor.

>> Try using one breath for the
leg float and another as the leg
returns to the floor.

>> Do ten on each leg, alternating
legs.

ATTENTION TO DETAIL *To maintain
pelvic alignment during the leg float,
place your fingertips under the hip
bones and be aware of feeling an even
pressure.*

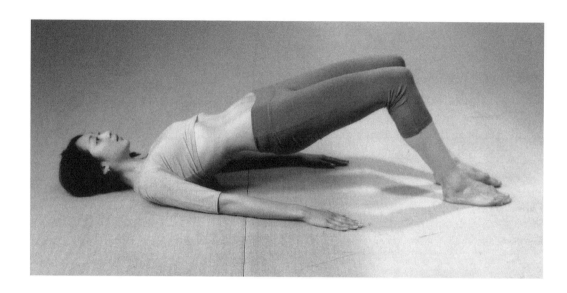

PELVIC PRESS ≫

This exercise strengthens the hamstrings.

≫ Align your bones in the supine position, palms facing down by your side.

≫ Starting with the tailbone, gradually peel the spine off the floor until just the shoulder blades are touching the floor.

≫ Keep the spine lengthened. Do not push up into an arch.

≫ Aim to bring the knee, hip and shoulder into alignment with each other. Reaching the kneecaps away from the hips can help achieve a lengthened connection between these areas.

≫ Feel the work through the hamstring and lower buttock muscles.

≫ Reverse the peeling action down toward the floor, with the tailbone being the last point to touch the floor. Be aware of articulating the vertebrae as you move the spine.

≫ Repeat.

ATTENTION TO DETAIL *Make sure you do not move the spine in an arch.*

ADVANCED
PELVIC PRESS »

>> Align your bones in the supine position, palms facing down.

>> Starting with the tailbone, gradually peel the spine off the floor until just the shoulder blades are touching the floor. Keep the spine lengthened. Do not push up into an arch.

>> Aim to bring the knee, hip and shoulder into alignment with each other.

>> Try not to clench the buttock muscles. Let them fall toward the knees.

>> Keeping the pelvis still, lift the foot and float one leg up and then return the foot to the floor.

>> Continue to alternate the leg floats while keeping the pelvis in the pelvic-press position. Don't do more than five times with each leg.

>> Reverse the original press back down to the floor, with the tailbone being the last point to touch the floor.

ATTENTION TO DETAIL *Be careful not to twist the hips.*

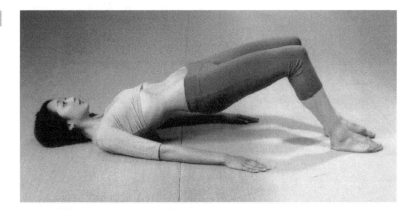

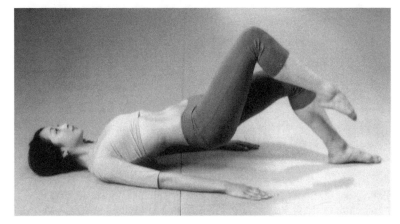

Suggested hamstring stretches

>> Beginner hamstring stretch, standing low (page 184).

>> Intermediate hamstring stretch, kneeling (page 186).

>> Advanced hamstring stretch, standing high (page 187).

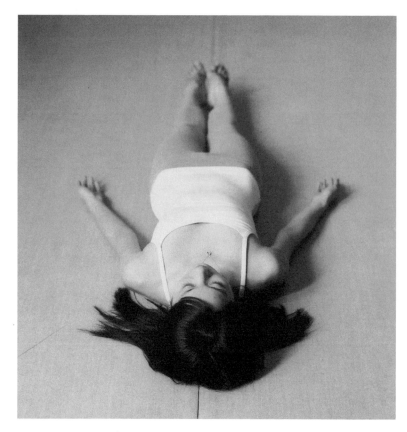

BUTTERFLY LEGS FOR THE HIPS AND INSIDE THIGH MUSCLES »

This exercise strengthens the muscles along the inside of the leg.

>> Align your bones in the supine position, with your arms down by your sides, palms facing up toward the ceiling.

>> Slide the legs out along the floor in front of you.

>> Gently rotate your legs outward but keep them together.

>> Reach your heel bones away from your sit bones to lengthen the legs.

>> Move the legs away from each other along the floor, to form a V, at a width that feels comfortable. Keep the pelvis still and aligned.

>> Bring the legs together and lightly press the heels together.

>> Repeat this ten times.

>> You should feel a sense of work through the inner legs, particularly as the heels press together.

ATTENTION TO DETAIL *Make sure the legs don't roll between inward and outward rotation.*

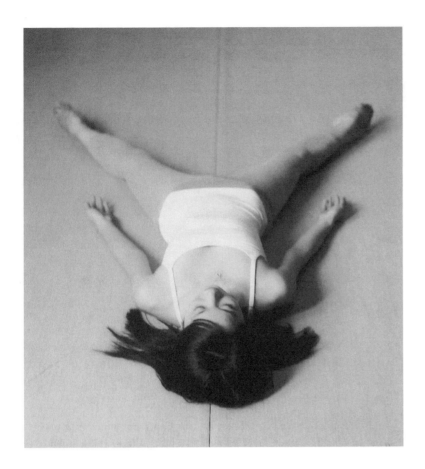

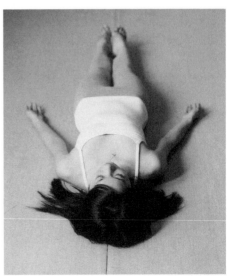

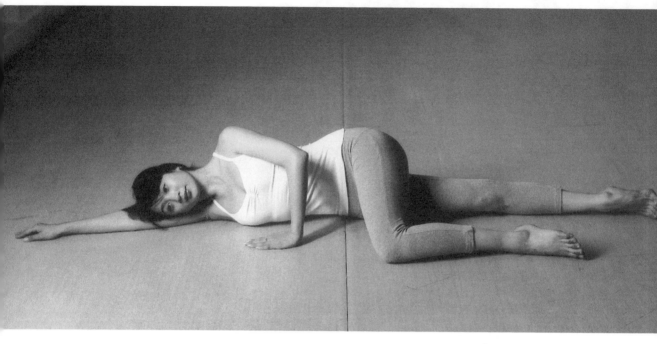

ALPHABET LEGS »

This exercise also strengthens the muscles along the inside of the leg.

» Align your bones in the side-lying position, with the top leg bent and the knee resting on the floor. Stretch the instep and flex the toes of the underneath leg.

» Reach the underneath heel away from your sit bones and raise the leg slightly off the floor.

» Begin to trace the letters of the alphabet in the air with the ball of your foot. It is important to keep the leg on the same level as your hip. Don't lower it to the floor.

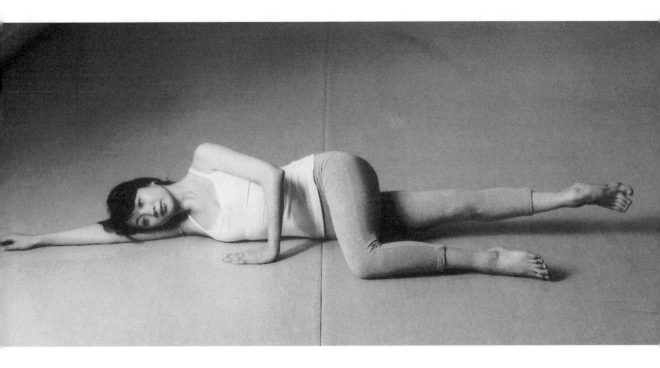

>> Try not to let the lifted leg rotate outward. Keep the back of the knee pointing toward the wall behind you.

>> Make sure your waist is lifted from the ground to maintain pelvic alignment.

>> Repeat the whole exercise to the other side.

ATTENTION TO DETAIL *Keep your waist lifted off the ground and the leg in parallel alignment.*

Suggested inside thigh stretches

» Inside thigh stretch on the wall in parallel alignment (page 182).

» Inside thigh stretch on the wall in outward rotation (page 183).

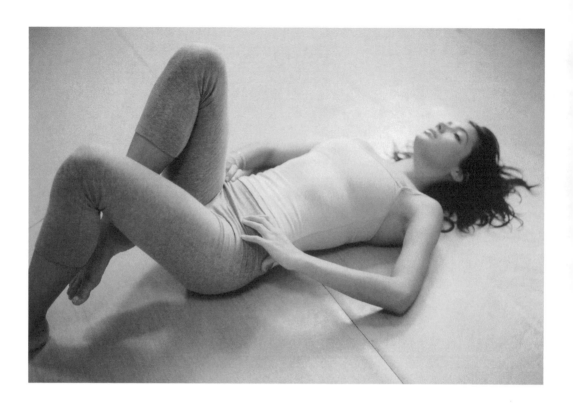

EVER-INCREASING
KNEE CIRCLES ≫

Explore a softening hip socket with this exercise. Feel the weight of the leg bone dropping into the pelvis.

≫ Align your bones in the supine position and float one leg up as in "knee circles for hips" on page 114.

≫ Begin to circle the thighbone at the hip joint either inward or outward by imagining that the kneecap is tracing small circles the size of a nickel.

≫ Allow the leg to cross the torso toward the pubic bone as the size of the knee circles increases.

≫ Begin to slowly increase the size of the circle to about the size of a dinner plate, without losing your pelvic alignment. As the size increases, allow the knee to fall slightly outward, bringing the leg into external rotation.

≫ Do ten circles in each direction, using one breath for each circle. Repeat with the other leg on the other side.

ATTENTION TO DETAIL *Keep the hip socket at the center of each circle.*

LEG CIRCLES >>

For this exercise you need to be able to extend the leg from the supine position up to 90 degrees comfortably, with no tightness in the back of the leg and without losing neutral pelvic alignment.

>> Align your bones in the supine position with your arms by your sides, palms facing up toward the ceiling.

>> Float one knee toward the chest and extend the leg and foot upward without tilting your sit bones to the ceiling. Allow the leg to softly rotate outward.

>> Begin to circle the leg at the hip joint by imagining the toe/heel is tracing circles the size of a nickel onto the ceiling.

>> Begin to slowly increase the size of the circle to about the size of a dinner plate without losing your pelvic alignment. As the circles become bigger allow the leg to externally rotate. Keep the bent knee pointing to the ceiling to stop the knee from wobbling.

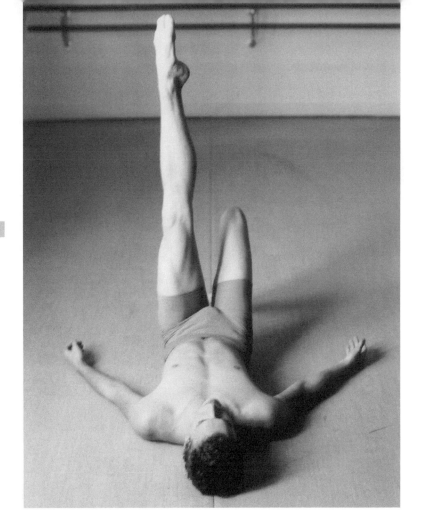

>> Keep your sit bones pointing to the wall in front of you.

>> Do ten circles in each direction, using one breath for each circle.

>> Repeat on the other side.

Suggested stretches

» Beginner iliopsoas, kneeling (page 188) or

» Advanced iliopsoas, lunging (page 189)

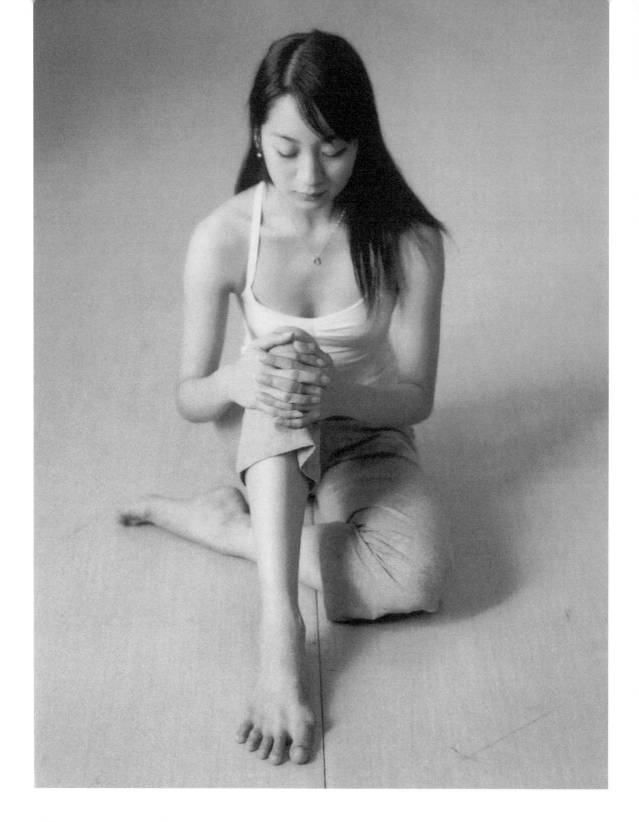

« ballet-fit workout »

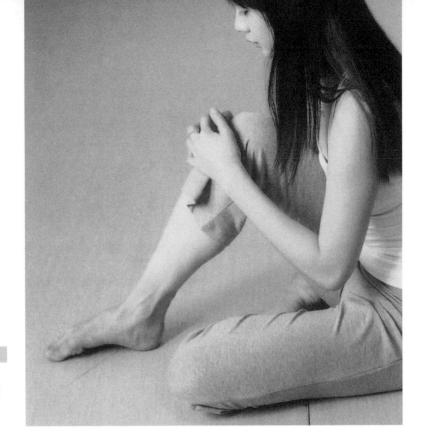

METATARSAL
PULL-UPS AND
TOE SPREADS »

This exercise is excellent if you spend a great deal of time in high-heeled shoes.

» It can be done sitting on the floor, as shown in the photograph, or sitting on a chair with both feet flat on the floor. It is best to use one foot at a time in this exercise.

» Spread the toes nice and wide on the floor.

» Now pull the metatarsals (the ball of the foot) up from the floor while keeping the toes and heel on the floor. Try to keep your toes flat and long as the center of the foot pulls up into a dome shape. This will be quite a small movement for most people. You should feel the work in the underside of your foot.

» Once the dome has reached its highest point, relax the foot back down to the floor and spread your toes nice and wide again. You have completed one pull-up. Make sure you work evenly across the toes. Don't pull toward the inside or outside of the foot as you pull the metatarsals up.

» Repeat this ten times on one foot before changing to the other foot.

ATTENTION TO DETAIL *Keep all five toes long and in contact with the floor. Remember not to roll to the inside or outside of the foot.*

EXTENSIONS AND FLEXIONS OF THE FOOT 》

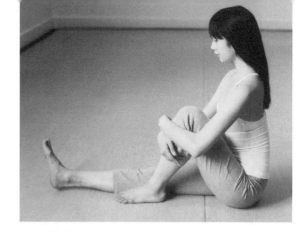

It is better to start with one foot at a time if you are new to this exercise.

》 It can be done sitting on the floor, as shown here, or with both legs extended in front of you in parallel alignment. Make sure the center of your knees, ankles and second toes are in alignment. Maintain this alignment.

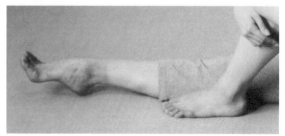

》 Gently flex the foot back toward you, toes pointing to the ceiling.

》 Keeping the toes flexed upward, reach the metatarsals (ball of foot) away from you and toward the floor. Imagine you are pushing the ball of your foot through soft, thick mud.

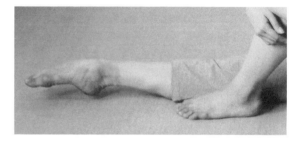

》 Continue this reaching action by pulling the toe bones long and away from the metatarsals.

》 Reverse the action back to a flexed foot. Take a breath for each direction.

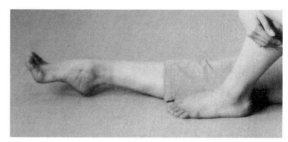

》 Do this ten times with the first foot and then change to the other foot.

》 You should feel work in the underside of the foot and a lengthening feeling through the whole leg.

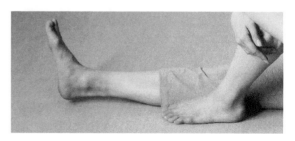

KNEE BENDS
IN PARALLEL »

The following three exercises develop the cornerstone of any dancer's technique: the demi-plié, which means "half-bend." We refer to it as a "knee bend." The knee bend begins, ends and links most movements in dance. It provides cushioning when landing from jumps, strengthens the legs, hips and back and gives rhythm to a dancer's movements.

>> Align your bones in the standing position. Focus directly ahead and maintain a lengthened spine and a broad back throughout this exercise.

>> Distribute your weight through the three points of each foot, with your center of gravity falling through the front of each ankle.

>> Bend the knees, keeping them on the vertical alignment in line with the second toe. Keep the sit bones pointing directly toward the floor.

>> Recover to the standing posture, feeling length at the front and back of the legs. If you have swayback legs, make sure you do not push back into the knees at the end of recovery.

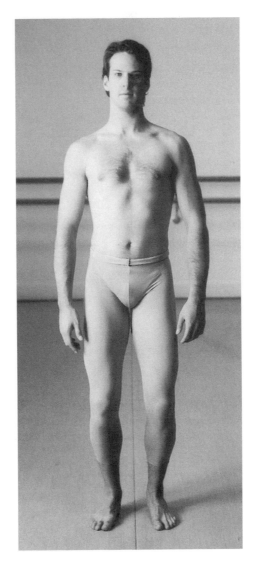

>> Repeat up to ten times. Try using one breath for each movement.

ATTENTION TO DETAIL *Alignment is crucial in knee bends. Remember to keep the knees on a vertical line with the second toe when working in parallel alignment and outward rotation.*

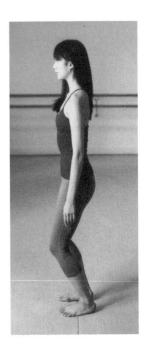

KNEE BENDS IN
OUTWARD ROTATION »

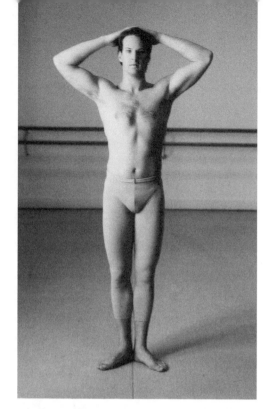

>> Align your bones in the standing position, with the legs and feet rotated outward to a point that feels comfortable—45 degrees is sufficient.

>> Place your hands on your head with the elbows gently pulling sideways, to feel a broadening across the back. Focus directly ahead and be aware of your alignment.

>> The thighbones should gently rotate outward throughout the exercise.

>> Lengthen the line between the heels and sit bones to help engage the inside thigh muscles.

>> Bend the knees in the direction of the second toe.

>> Keep your sit bones pointing directly toward the floor and imagine them widening as you go down. Everyone has varying depths of knee bends, as you can see in the difference between the two dancers in the photographs.

>> Recover to a standing position.

>> Repeat up to ten times. Try using one breath for each movement.

ATTENTION TO DETAIL *Imagine the knees escaping from each other and enjoy the feeling of moving with gravity. Maintain a lengthened spine.*

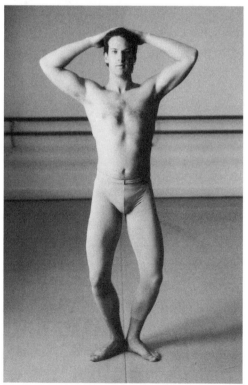

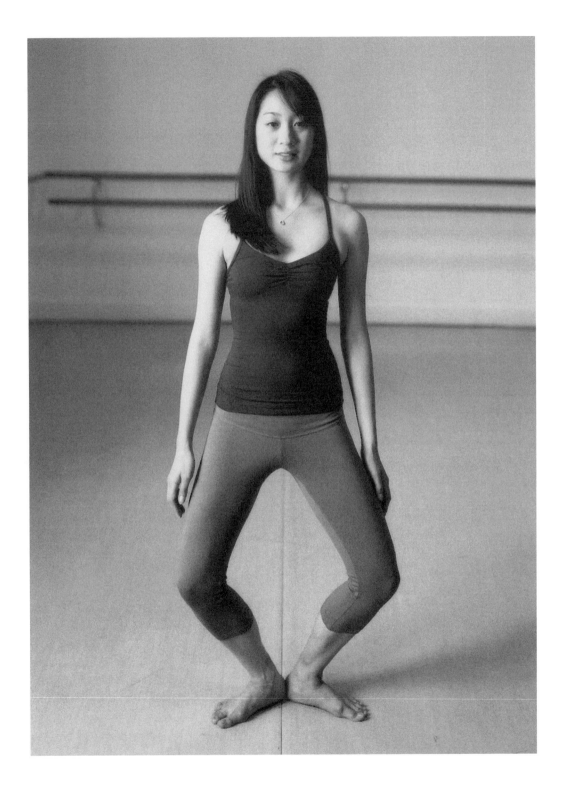

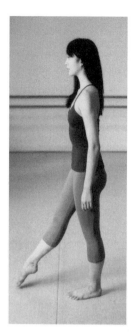

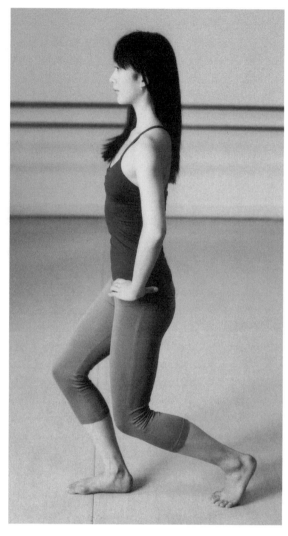

FORWARD
WEIGHT
TRANSFER >>

This exercise strengthens
the muscles of the knee.

>> Align your bones in the standing
position, with your arms by the
sides or your hands on your hips.

>> Slide the right foot forward along
the floor and as it stretches allow
it to lift off the floor.

>> Step forward, transferring your
weight onto the right leg, with the
knee bending in line with the
second toe, until the left foot
releases from the floor. As your
weight falls into the right leg,
make sure the right knee is
in line with the second toe.

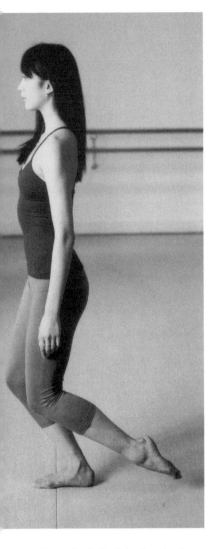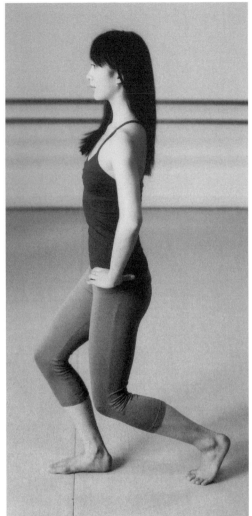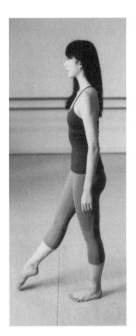

>> Place the ball of the foot back on the floor and reverse the movement by stepping backward onto the left leg to the beginning posture.

>> Repeat up to ten times on the right leg and then on the left leg.

ATTENTION TO DETAIL *Maintain a lengthened spine, with your sit bones directed down toward the floor. Make sure your hips have not twisted. Keep them level.*

Suggested stretches

» Standing thigh stretch (page 190).

» Advanced thigh stretch (page 193).

SIDEWAYS WEIGHT TRANSFERS »

The goal of this exercise is to maintain a neutral pelvis and level hips.

» Align your bones in the standing position, with feet and legs slightly rotated outward and slightly apart. Put your hands on your hips and use your fingers to monitor the activity of the oblique muscles.

» Transfer all your weight onto the right leg, releasing the left heel, but maintain the contact with the floor through the ball of the left foot.

» Return slowly through the starting position and then move to the other side. Work with a feeling of length through the legs. If you have swayback legs, be careful not to lock the knees backward as you transfer the weight onto them.

» Do up to ten transfers on each side.

ATTENTION TO DETAIL *Keep the hips level on the horizontal plane as you move and keep the oblique muscles soft. Keeping the hips still and on the horizontal plane will stimulate the deep abdominal muscles.*

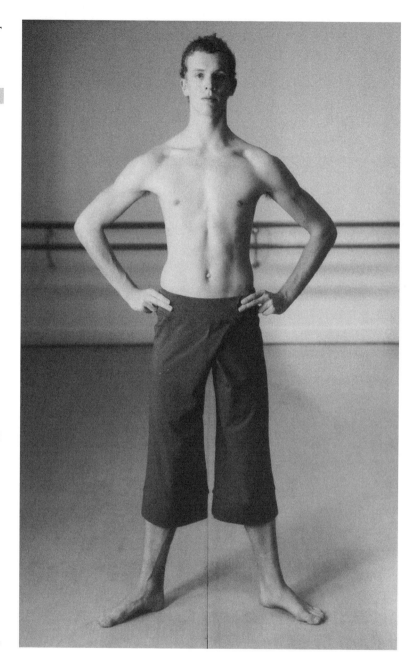

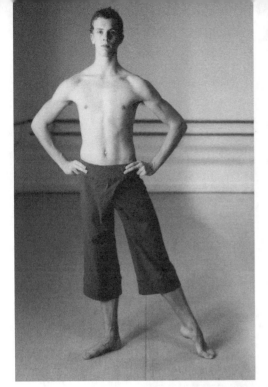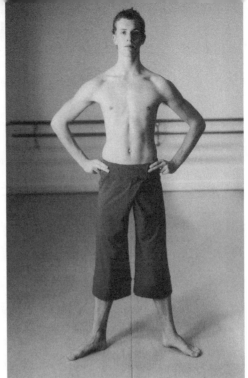

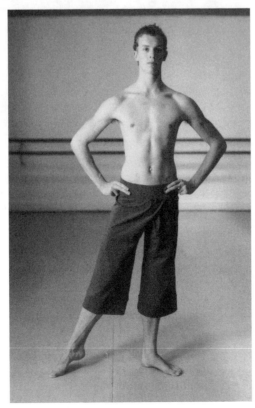

CALF RAISES IN PARALLEL ON TWO FEET >>

This exercise develops endurance in the calf muscles.

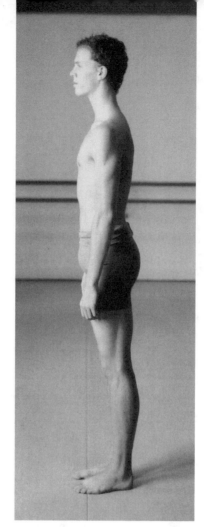
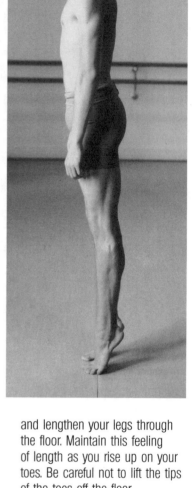

>> Align your bones in the standing position. You can rest your hands on the back of a chair for extra support.

>> Distribute your weight through the three points of each foot, with your center of gravity falling through the front of each ankle. Feel length through the front and back of the leg.

>> Without leaning forward or backward, feel the crown of your head reaching to the ceiling and lengthen your legs through the floor. Maintain this feeling of length as you rise up on your toes. Be careful not to lift the tips of the toes off the floor.

>> As you lower the heels back down to the floor, imagine leaving your head where it is and feel length through the body.

>> Repeat ten times.

CALF RAISES IN PARALLEL ON ONE FOOT »

These raises are the same as those performed on two legs, but with one foot placed by the inside of the ankle bone on the other leg.

» Align your bones in the standing position and place the toes of your left foot on the inside of your right ankle bone. You can rest your hands on the back of a chair for extra support.

» Distribute your weight through the three points of the foot, with your center of gravity falling through the front of the ankle. Feel length through the front and back of the leg.

» Without leaning forward or backward, feel the crown of your head reaching to the ceiling and lengthen your legs through the floor.

» Rise up on your toes. Keep the tips of your toes flat on the floor.

» Do the single leg raises until you feel your calf muscle beginning to tire.

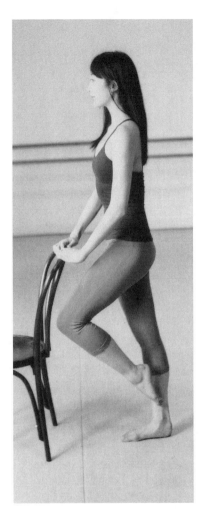

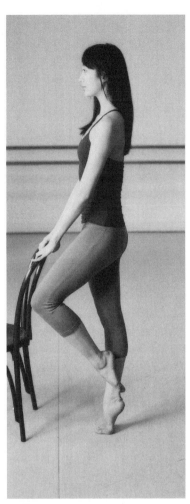

» Try to do the same number of raises on each leg. If one leg is weaker, build the number of repetitions on the weaker leg to match the stronger one, and then increase the number evenly on both sides. Slowly build the number of raises over time: 25 to 35 is an adequate result for an active person. Maintain this level by doing your raises regularly.

Suggested stretches

» Lunging calf stretch (page 200).

» Kneeling Achilles (page 201).

PRANCES IN PARALLEL ALIGNMENT, INWARD AND OUTWARD ROTATIONS >>

This exercise mobilizes internal and external rotation of the hips. Prances should feel loose and light. Make sure your knees are over your second toes in all the bends.

ATTENTION TO DETAIL *During all the prances try to keep the hips still and level on the horizontal line. Make sure that the inward and outward rotations are within your comfort range.*

>> Align your bones in the standing position. Place your hands on your hips and extend one foot off the floor, toes pointing down, and bend the leg you are standing on.

>> Gently push up through a rise on the standing leg and drop onto the foot that is raised. This is one prance.

>> Continue transferring the weight from one foot to the other in parallel alignment for up to 20 prances. Develop a momentum and keep moving.

>> Now continue, doing up to 20 prances into an inward rotation by turning the thighs, knees and feet in toward the pubic bone.

>> Continue the prances into parallel alignment for up to 20 prances.

>> Now continue, doing up to 20 more prances into outward rotation by opening the knees to the side.

>> Return to parallel alignment for a final series of up to 20 prances.

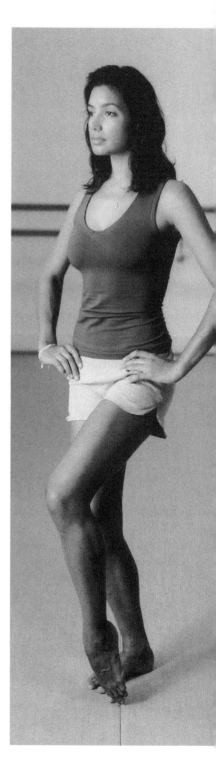

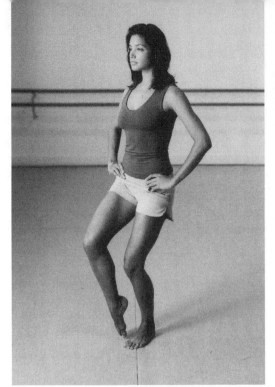

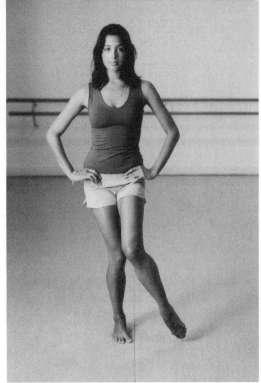

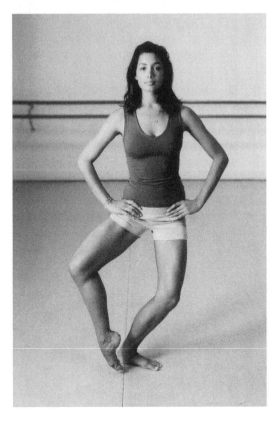

alignm

dynamic

rebal

awarenes

>> the arm ar

back

holistic

ent
stability
ncing
ds
d
connection
balance

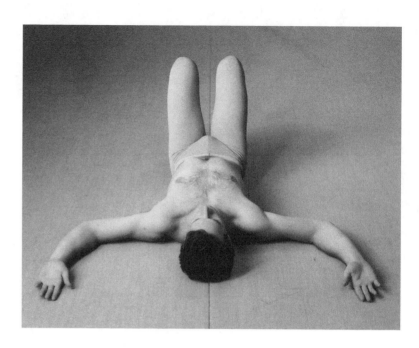

CHICKEN WINGS >>

This exercise opens the chest and strengthens the muscles that stabilize the shoulder blades. The back should feel nice and broad. Chicken wings can also be done sitting or standing. If your arms rest easily on the ground, lay the spine (including tailbone and head) on a tightly rolled up beach towel to increase the intensity of the exercise.

>> Align your bones in the supine position, with the arms bent to the sides, making a 90-degree angle, elbows in line with shoulders.

>> Slide the arms along the floor toward your head, with your hands moving toward each other.

>> Initiate the return by pulling the elbows sideways, away from the shoulders, as the arms slide back to the beginning position.

>> Make sure the shoulder blades are wide and do not dig into the floor.

>> Repeat ten times.

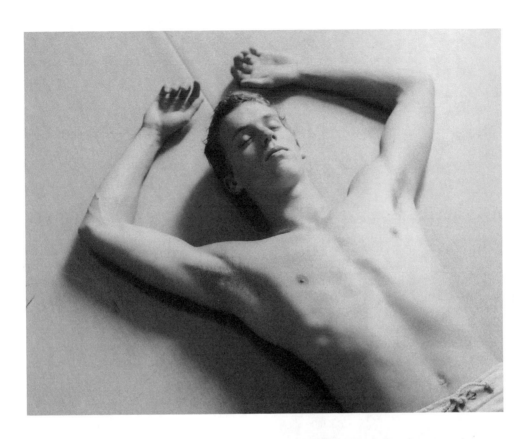

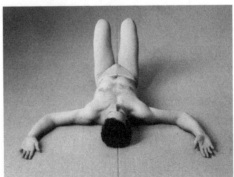

ZIG-ZAG ARMS ≫

This exercise develops shoulder stability. You may find it helpful to do it one arm at a time, with your head turned to check the alignment.

≫ Align your bones in the prone position, with arms bent and elbows in line with your shoulders and reaching sideways. Your palms should be flat and facing the floor. You can rest your head to one side or rest your forehead on the floor.

≫ Lift the forearm from the floor, keeping the elbow lightly touching the floor.

≫ Now lift the elbow from the ground but keep the hand higher than the elbow. Be careful not to bend or twist the wrist.

≫ Return the elbow to the ground, then the forearm and then the hand. Repeat up to five times with one arm before moving to the other side.

≫ Try using one breath for each movement and keep the back broad and wide.

ATTENTION TO DETAIL *Zig-zag arms can be an intense exercise. Don't overdo it. Work on building up over a few weeks.*

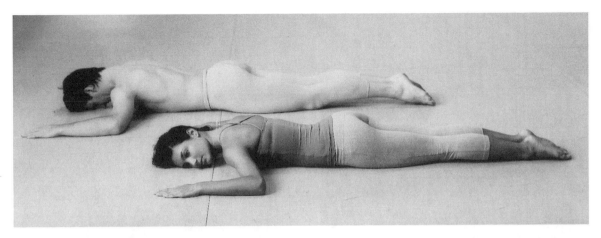

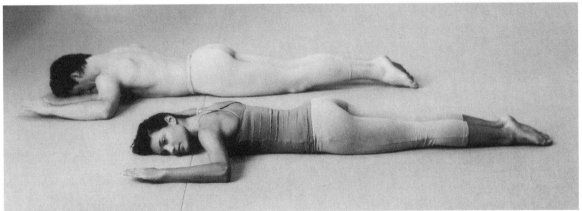

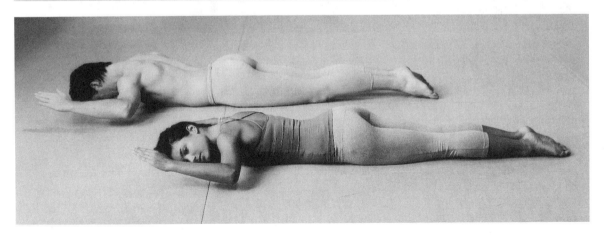

DOUBLE ARM FLOATS >>

Use this exercise to explore your full range of arm movements while your neutral spine alignment is supported by contact with the floor.

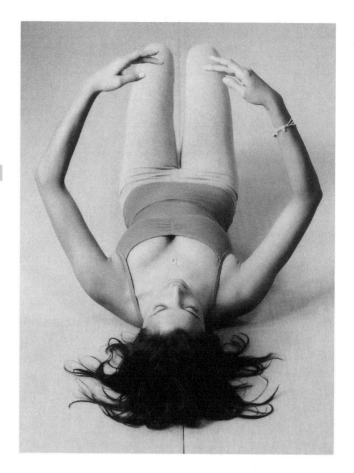

>> Align your bones in the supine posture, palms facing up toward the ceiling, arms by your side.

>> Gently feel the shoulder blades pull flat and wide as you lift both arms toward the ceiling to hold an imaginary giant ball. The palms should face slightly toward your breastbone and the elbows should soften sideways. This is the front position.

>> Feel the weight of the arm bones falling into the shoulder joints and feel these joints falling through the floor.

>> Keep hold of the imaginary ball and move your arms so that the palms of your hands face the crown of your head and your elbows face out to each side. This is the high position.

>> Without letting your arms drop toward the floor, reach them sideways until they are just below the top of your shoulders, elbows soft and pointing toward the floor, with the forearms and hands continuing the curved line. Reach the elbows away from the body. This is the side position.

>> Bring your arms toward each other to the front position, with the feeling of hugging a huge tree, to complete the first arm float.

>> Use a breath to move to each arm position and then build up to one breath for each arm float.

>> Do this up to ten times.

ATTENTION TO DETAIL *Watch that you don't lose the flatness of the shoulder blades or close in across the chest. Try to relax and let the arm drop into the socket throughout the exercise.*

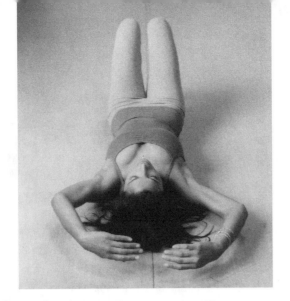

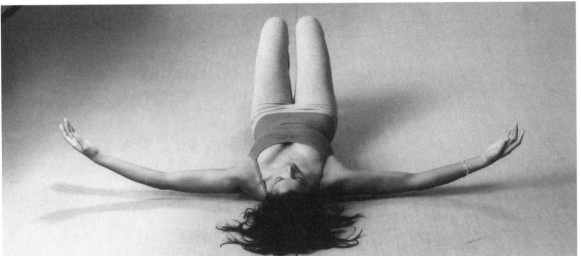

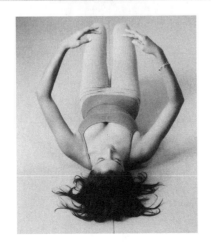

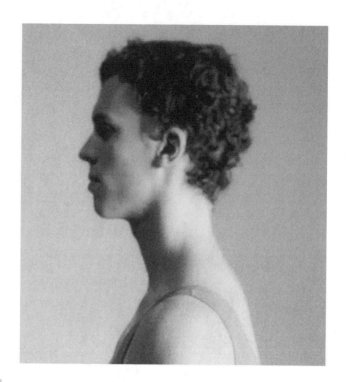

CHIN TUCKS ≫

This exercise strengthens the muscles at the front of the neck. It is particularly good if you unconsciously poke your head forward while working at a computer for long periods.

≫ Sit on a chair and align your bones in the sitting position.

≫ Gently pull the chin back into the neck without dropping your face toward the floor. Imagine you're making a double chin!

≫ Be careful not to disturb the shoulders.

≫ Release the chin.

≫ Repeat up to ten times.

ATTENTION TO DETAIL *This photo shows good length and alignment through the neck.*

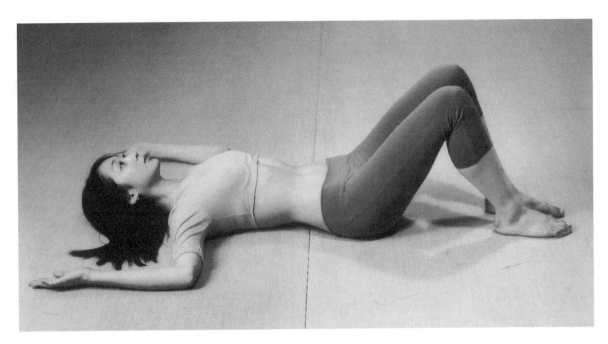

NOSE CIRCLES 〉〉

This exercise helps to release neck and jaw tension. For improved comfort, place a small, folded towel under your head. It can also be done sitting, with your back against a wall. You can even do nose circles against the headrest in your car while waiting at traffic lights.

〉〉 Align your bones in the supine position. Close your eyes and breathe naturally.

〉〉 Relax the muscles of the face and feel the base of the skull resting heavily into the floor. Let the chin fall softly toward the neck.

〉〉 Trace small circles the size of a nickel with the tip of your nose.

〉〉 Continue this for 60 seconds clockwise and then repeat counterclockwise.

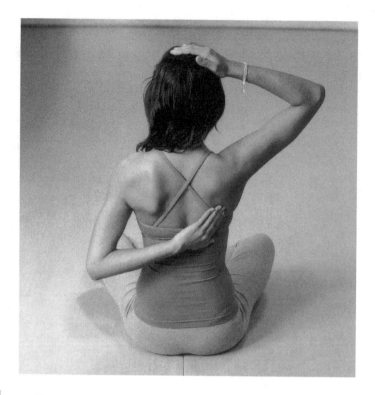

SINGLE ARM
FLOATS, SITTING >>

The intention of the next three exercises is to move the arms while keeping the shoulder-blades wide and flat. You can use one hand to check your shoulder alignment, as shown in the photograph, or you can ask a friend to place a thumb near the shoulder blade tip to help your kinetic awareness.

>> Align your bones in the sitting position on the floor or a chair, with one hand on your head and one checking your shoulder blade alignment.

>> Take your hand from your head to the high position, with the palm facing the crown of the head and the elbow pointing out to the side.

>> Move the arm sideways into the side position just below shoulder height, with your elbow facing behind you and your palm facing the front. Keep a gentle curve through the whole arm, reaching out sideways from the back.

>> Bring the arm across and down to the front position, with your hand opposite your belly button. Keep the shoulder blade alignment and imagine hugging a huge tree. Keep your chest open and your back broadening.

>> Lift the arm up to the high position to begin another arm float.

>> Repeat five arm floats in total, checking the shoulder blade with the other hand, and five times without this contact. Repeat on the other side.

ATTENTION TO DETAIL *Imagine you have a space between each vertebra to lengthen the natural curves of the spine.*

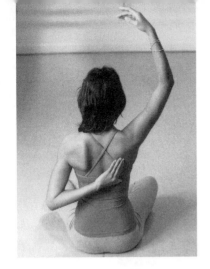

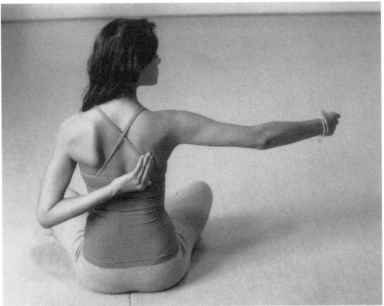

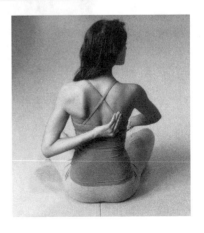

DOUBLE ARM
FLOATS, SITTING »

» Align your bones in the sitting position on the floor or a chair. Same as for single arm floats but use two arms instead.

» Do this up to ten times.

ATTENTION TO DETAIL *Feel each arm movement radiating outward from the spine, across the shoulder blades and along each arm to the fingertips.*

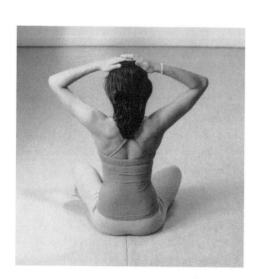

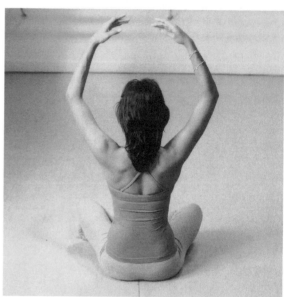

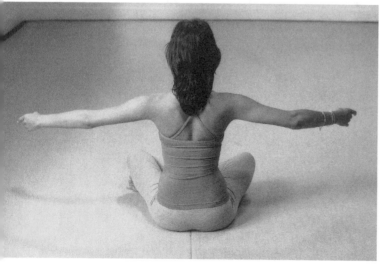

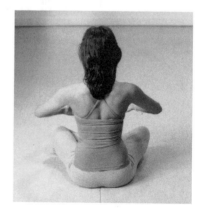

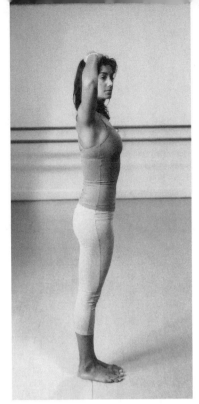

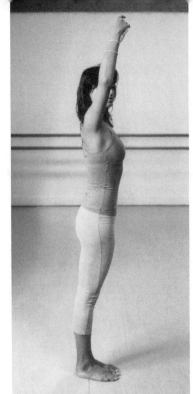

DOUBLE ARM FLOATS, STANDING »

>> Align your bones in the standing position.

>> Use two arms at the same time.

>> Watch yourself sideways in a mirror to check your alignment. For added difficulty, you can add this exercise to any leg work such as weight transfers from the "From Hips to Toes" section. This will help develop your whole-body coordination.

ATTENTION TO DETAIL *Maintain a sense of broadness across the back.*

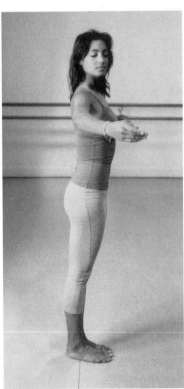

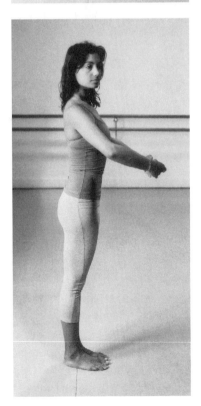

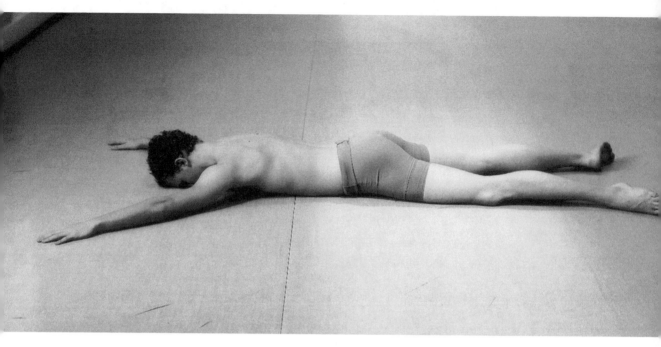

ALTERNATING ARM REACH »

This exercise isolates movement in the arm socket to help create a stable shoulder girdle.

» Align your bones in the prone position, making a V shape with the arms and legs. Feel broad across your back.

» Have your palms facing the floor. Very slightly, rotate the left arm so the elbow falls toward the floor.

» Reach the arm along the floor until it lifts slightly.

» Try to feel a connection between the left shoulder blade and the right hip.

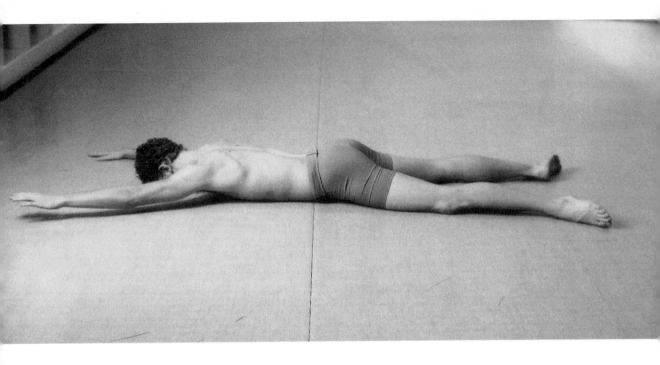

>> Keep the spine long and be
careful not to arch your back.

>> Return the arm to the floor.

>> Repeat with alternating arms
up to five times on each side

ATTENTION TO DETAIL *Keep the*
shoulder blades broadening during the
movement and maintain space between
the shoulder and the ear.

FOUR-POINT
PUSH-UPS »

This exercise works the triceps and tones the underarm region very effectively. Move only as far as you can, maintain alignment and build up slowly. One good push-up is worth a hundred poor ones.

» Align your bones in the four-point kneeling position, with the shoulder blade tips toward your armpits, broadening your back. Create length from your ears to your shoulders.

» Bend your elbows down toward the floor. It is important to keep the elbows from moving out to the side and to hinge from the hips.

» For the first few push-ups, turn your head to the side and observe your spine and shoulders in a mirror. Keep the spine long and neutral and try to maintain a lengthened neck. Be careful not to lift the chin.

» Stop just above the floor and then return to the starting position.

» Try using one breath for each direction of movement and over time build up to ten push-ups.

ATTENTION TO DETAIL *Push-ups require correct shoulder, spine and pelvic alignment to be effective.*

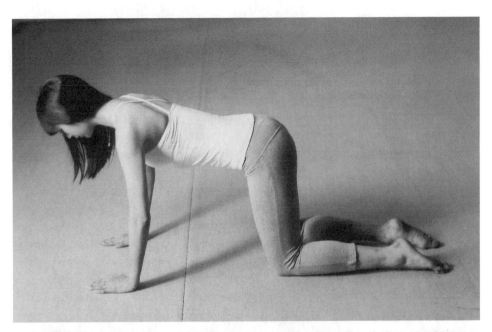

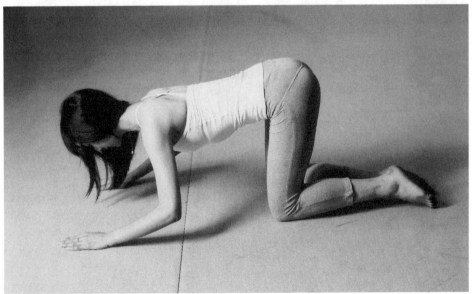

FULL PUSH-UPS >>

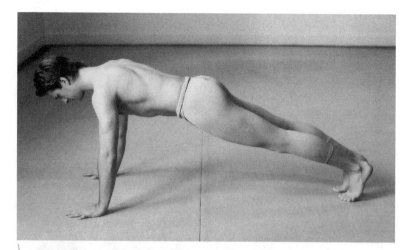

When you are confident with your push-up technique, throw these exercises into a warm-up to get the upper body and arms going.

>> Align your bones in the four-point kneeling position and extend both legs behind you into the traditional push-up shape. Lengthen your toes and press into the floor evenly.

>> Bend your elbows down toward the floor. It is important to keep the elbows from moving out to the side and to hinge from the hips.

>> For the first few push-ups, turn your head to the side and observe your spine and shoulders in a mirror. Keep the spine long and neutral and try to maintain a lengthened neck. Be careful not to lift the chin and shorten the back of the neck. By paying detailed attention to your shoulder alignment and spinal/pelvic alignment during these push-ups you will experience a fuller workout for the shoulder girdle and arms.

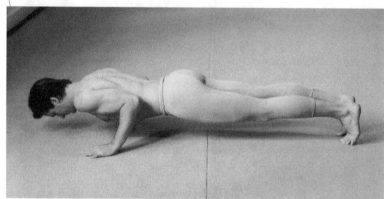

>> Stop just above the floor and then return to the starting position, or take it to a comfortable distance from the floor, where good alignment can be maintained.

>> Once you have mastered the alignment and worked the full arm range, build up to completing ten full push-ups, using one breath for each push-up.

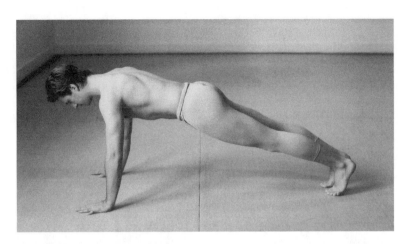

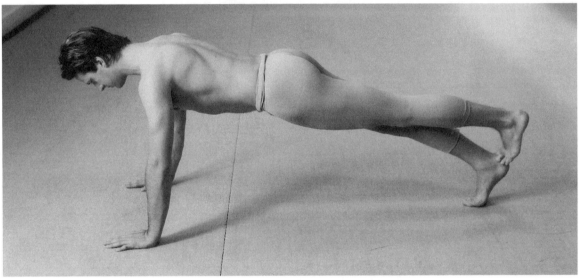

FULL PUSH-UPS, ONE-LEGGED »

» Align your bones in the four-point kneeling position and extend both legs behind you into the traditional push-up shape, or take it to a comfortable distance from the floor, where good alignment can be maintained.

» Place the toes of the left foot on to the right heel.

» Proceed exactly as for full push-ups, maintaining a lengthened spine, particularly the lower spine, and keep the pelvis level on the horizontal alignment.

» Build to ten push-ups, using one breath for each push-up.

align

dynami

rebal

awaren

>>lengthen

holisti

and release

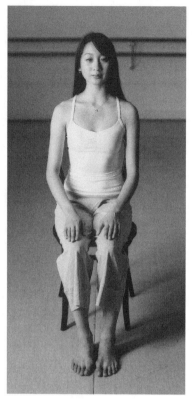
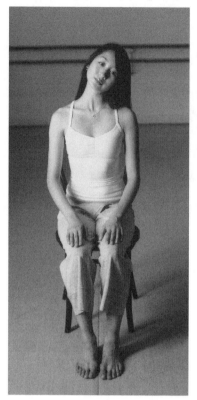
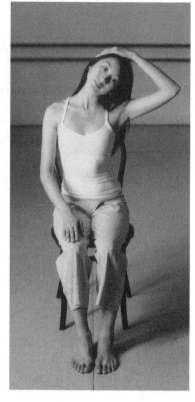

The stretches in this section suit a range of abilities, from a less active person to a professional dancer. Be sure to do the ones most appropriate for you.

SIDEWAYS NECK STRETCH »

These exercises relieve neck and upper back tension.

» Align your bones in the sitting position on a chair. Focus your eyes straight ahead.

» Let your left ear fall to your left shoulder.

» Place the left fingertips on your right ear and allow them to act as a weight. Do not pull.

» Maintain even pressure through your sit bones.

» Hold for ten breaths, return and repeat on the other side.

ATTENTION TO DETAIL *Use natural breathing and relax into the stretches. Don't force the stretch.*

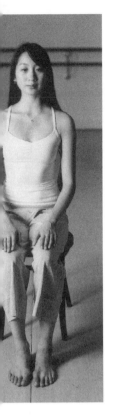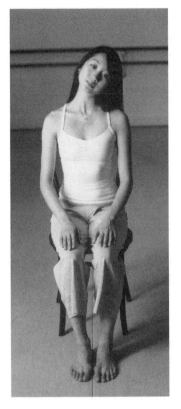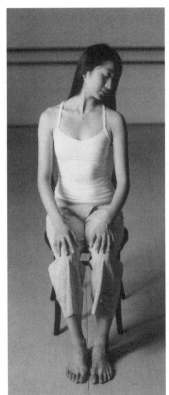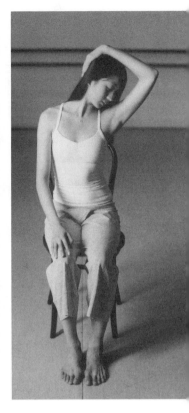

DIAGONAL
NECK STRETCH »

>> Align your bones in the sitting position on a chair. Focus your eyes straight ahead.

>> Let your left ear fall to your left shoulder.

>> Turn your head toward your left shoulder, taking the eye focus down toward the floor.

>> Place the left fingertips on the back of your head and allow them to act as a weight. Do not pull.

>> Hold for ten breaths, return and repeat on the other side.

OPENING
THE CHEST »

You can increase the stretch across the chest by placing a rolled-up towel between the shoulder blades under the spine. This exercise is excellent for nursing mothers.

>> Align your bones in the supine position, with the arms open and bent at a 90-degree angle on the floor, just above the shoulders. Feel your bones fall through the floor.

>> If your elbows or hands do not touch the floor, place a small towel under them and gradually remove it during the exercise.

>> Let your chin fall softly toward the throat. Listen to your breath.

>> Gently pull the elbows away from the shoulders.

>> Stay in this position for several minutes, relaxing and breathing.

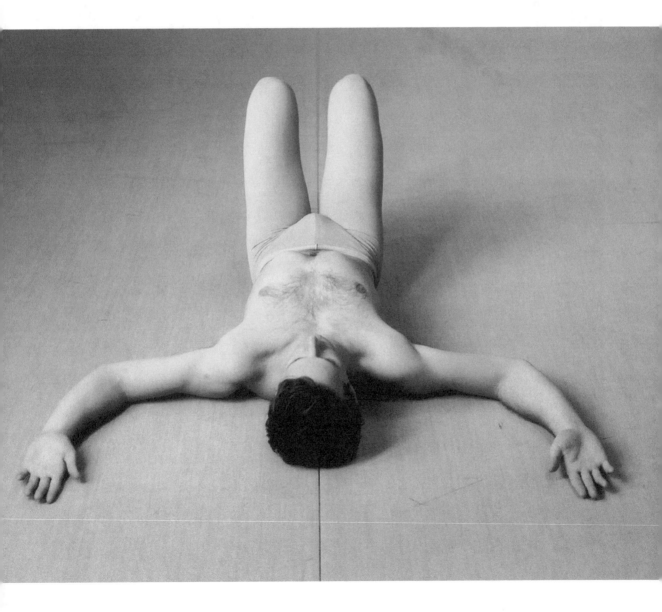

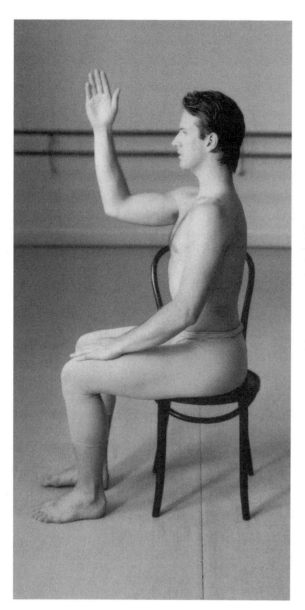
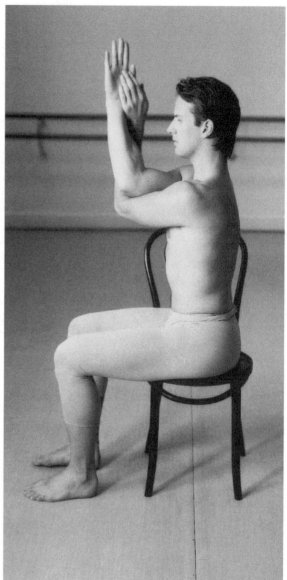

« ballet-fit workout »

UPPER ARM
AND SHOULDER
STRETCH »

This stretch helps to release shoulder and back tension.

» Align your bones in the sitting position on a chair. Keep the spine lengthening throughout the exercise.

» Bend the right arm up in front of you with the elbow at shoulder height and the inside of your arm facing sideways away from your face.

» Slide the left arm under the right and try to bring the palms together. For those who can't reach up to keep palms together —hold a small towel or Elastic exercise band. Keep the elbows at shoulder height, with fingers pointing to the ceiling.

» Allow the neck and shoulders to relax.

» Hold for up to ten breaths or 60 seconds.

» Unfold the arms and repeat on the other side.

STRETCHING THE CHEST MUSCLES WITH A HAND ON THE WALL »

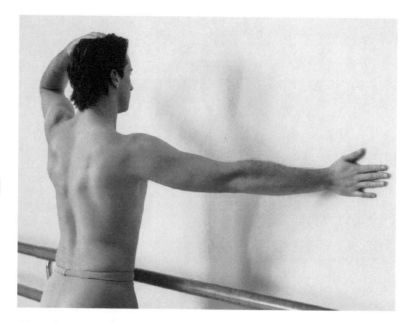

This stretch opens up the chest.

» Align your bones in the standing posture, facing a wall and about one foot away. Being closer to the wall will make the stretch more intense.

» Stretch out your arm. Place your right palm level with your shoulder on the wall and your left hand on your head. Pull the right shoulder blade tip wide.

» Maintain your spinal alignment and walk on the spot, turning your body to the left away from the wall, leaving the right arm and hand behind on the wall. The movement occurs in the arm. Keep the shoulder blade as flat and wide as possible. If you find that your shoulder blade slides into the spine as you turn, take your body slightly toward the wall as you turn.

» You should feel a gentle stretch across the right side of your chest in front of the shoulder.

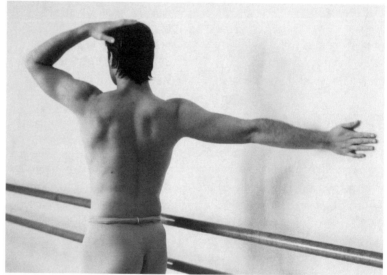

» Hold this position for up to ten deep breaths, keeping the neck and shoulders relaxed.

» Turn back to the starting position and repeat on the other side.

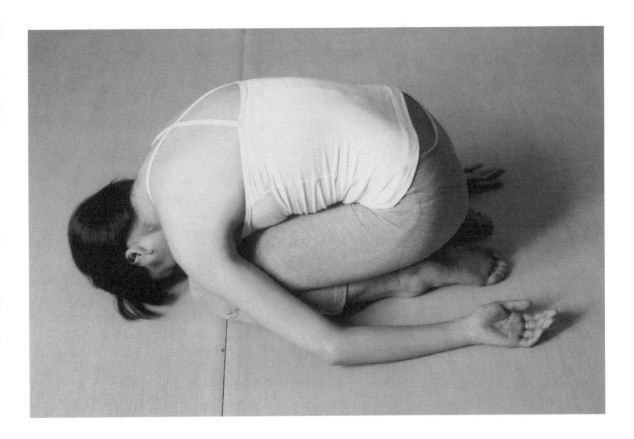

CHILD'S POSE »

This is a gentle stretch for the lower back and a great resting place to calm the mind and body.

» Kneel on the floor and bend your body forward from the hips. Rest your forehead on the ground and let your arms fall to the side of the body with your palms facing up toward the ceiling. If you don't like your knees being in a tight bend, you may prefer to place a rolled-up towel between the lower and upper legs.

» Feel your whole body relax and soften. Let your bones fall into each other and through the floor. Stay in this position for a few minutes. Observe the natural rhythm of the breath.

LOWER BACK AND SIDE STRETCH FOR BEGINNERS »

This exercise releases tension around the ribs and lower back.

» Align the bones in the sitting position on the floor with the legs crossed.

» Take one arm above your head, reaching the fingers to the ceiling. Rest the back of the other hand on your thigh.

» Reach the torso up and over as you bend sideways toward the hand resting on your thigh, reaching the arm diagonally up toward the ceiling. Use the other hand to support the body from falling forward in front of the legs.

» Strongly reach your sit bones directly down into the floor to work the stretch into the side and back muscles. If you can only feel this stretch in the side of the body, tilt your sit bones slightly toward the knees, creating a small C curve in the lower back, to move the stretch into the lower back muscles. Do this only once when you are in the stretch. There should be no lower back pain.

» Don't let the hip opposite to the direction of the stretch come in front of the other hip on the stretched side.

» Imagine that the chest is spiraling up to the ceiling as you lengthen your torso out of the pelvis.

» Hold this stretch for up to ten breaths and return to the starting position by reversing the actions. Repeat on the other side.

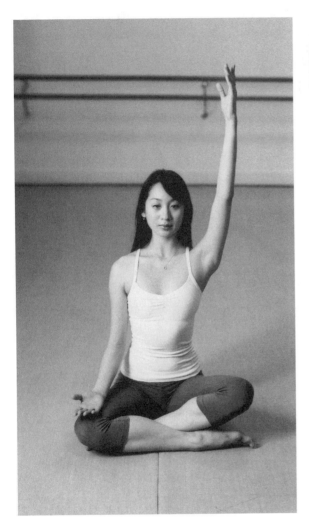
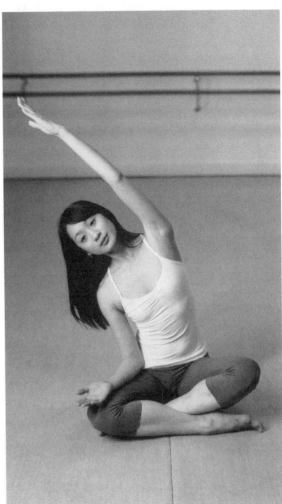

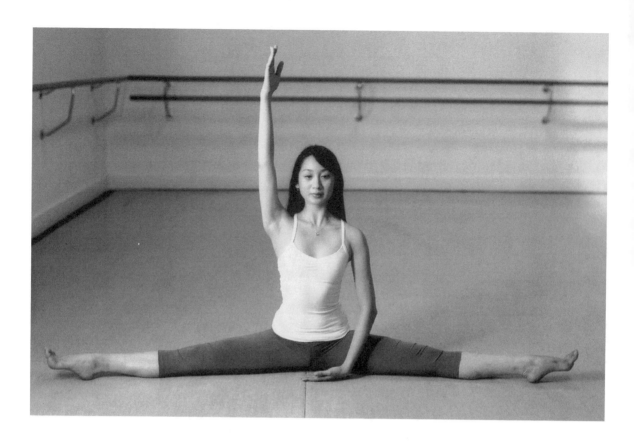

ADVANCED LOWER BACK AND SIDE STRETCH »

This stretch takes time to master and requires small lengthening movements in the torso to move the stretch through the side of the torso and into the back. As you breathe, relax the areas where you feel the stretch and feel them lengthening.

» Align your bones in the sitting position on the floor, with your legs open to the side as far as is comfortable. Maintain your spinal alignment and keep the knees facing up toward the ceiling. Extend the ankles and flex the toes up toward the ceiling.

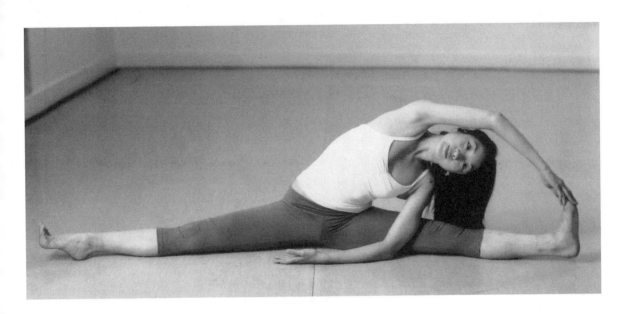

>> Take one arm above your head and reach the fingers to the ceiling. Place the other hand on the floor in front of you, palm facing up.

>> Reach your torso up and over as you bend sideways until you can hold your foot. Let the other elbow rest on the ground and use it to support you and stop you from falling forward. If you can't reach your foot just leave your arm by your ear.

>> Strongly reach your sit bones directly down into the floor to work the stretch into the side and back muscles.

>> Imagine that the chest is spiraling up to the ceiling as you lengthen the torso out of the pelvis and along the leg.

>> Hold this stretch for up to ten breaths and return to the starting posture by reversing the actions. Repeat on the other side.

« lengthen and release »

175

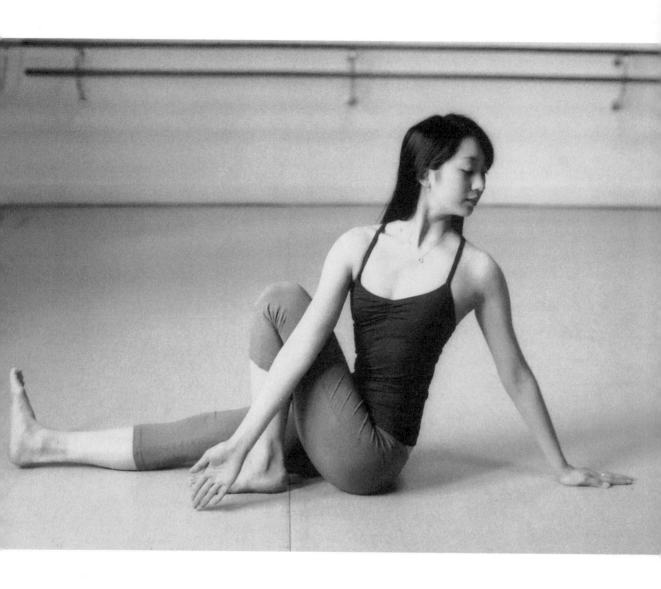

« ballet-fit workout »

SPINAL SPIRAL >>

This exercise stretches the back through rotation and relieves back tension and clears the mind.

>> Align your bones in the cross-legged sitting position on the floor, with your legs extended in front of you.

>> Bend the left knee and place the heel close to your left sit bone.

>> Place the left hand on the floor behind you in line with your left hip.

>> Slide and reach the right arm and hand in front of the left knee, toward the floor. Look over the right shoulder. Keep the fingers of the right hand reaching into the floor.

>> Reach the right heel away from right sit bone.

>> Lengthen the spine and spiral to the left.

>> Keep the left knee pointing to the ceiling throughout the exercise.

>> Imagine that your sit bones are roots growing strongly into the ground to maintain pelvic alignment.

>> Do this for ten breaths.

>> Repeat on the other side.

EASY CROSS-LEGS FOR BUTTOCK MUSCLES »

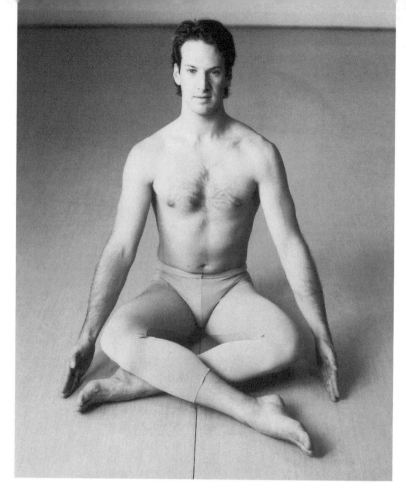

This stretch relieves lower back and hip tension.

>> Align the bones in the cross-legged sitting position and slightly overcross the legs.

>> Place the hands by the knees with fingertips pointing toward the floor.

>> Drop your torso forward over the legs, slide and reach your hands forward into a V shape.

>> Press the hands lightly into the floor with your palms facing each other. At the same time, reach your tailbone down into the floor behind you.

>> Relax the front of your hips as they fold and crease.

>> Hold the position for ten breaths.

>> Recover, rolling up through a curved spine, articulating each vertebra, and change the crossover of the legs to repeat on the other side.

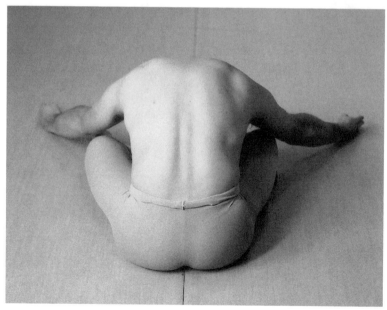

ADVANCED BUTTOCK MUSCLE STRETCH »

This stretch requires iliopsoas, adductor and hamstring flexibility.

» Align your bones in a cross-legged sitting position. Bend the right leg in front at a 45-degree angle and extend the left leg behind the left hip in parallel alignment.

» Place the left hand on the front ankle and the right hand on the knee.

» Keep both hips facing the wall in front of you and not twisting back toward the extended leg. You should feel a stretch through the buttock muscle of the bent leg.

» Hold for five breaths to begin with. Over time build up to ten breaths or 60 seconds.

» To intensify the stretch move the sit bone of the bent leg along the ground and sideways toward the front heel.

ATTENTION TO DETAIL *Make sure the front bent knee is parallel to the hips. This is an extremely advanced stretch. Do not attempt it if you are in any doubt.*

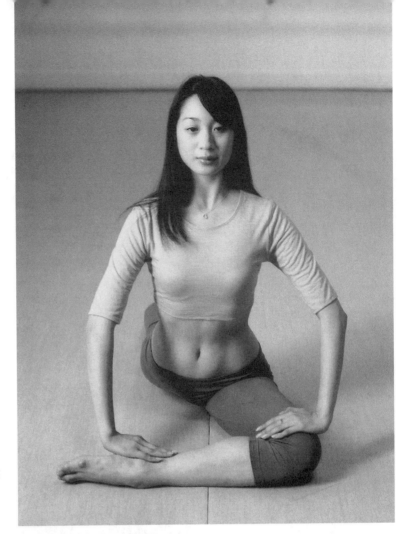

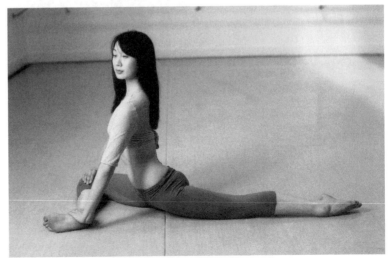

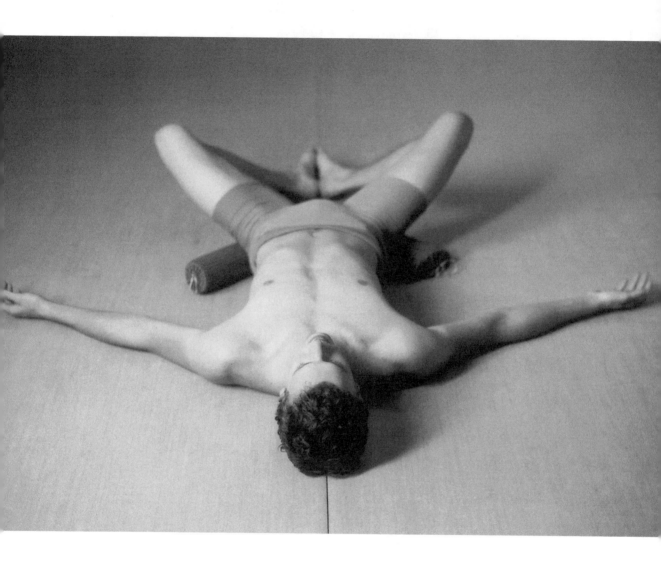

FROGS FOR THE
HIP MUSCLES >>

This exercise gently stretches the inside of the thighs and the pelvic region.

>> Align the bones in the supine position, with your arms stretched sideways, palms facing up toward the ceiling.

>> Drop one knee at a time to the floor to make the frog position. Keep the soles of the feet together.

>> Place cushions or pillows under the upper thighs to provide extra support. You can remove them as you become more flexible.

>> You should feel relaxed.

>> Keep your sit bones parallel to the floor. Do not lift them up toward the ceiling.

ATTENTION TO DETAIL *Do not press the legs down to the floor. Let gravity do the work.*

INSIDE THIGH STRETCH ON THE WALL IN PARALLEL ALIGNMENT >>

For this exercise you need to be able to extend the leg from the supine position up to 90 degrees comfortably, with no tightness in the back of the leg and without losing the neutral pelvic alignment.

>> Align the bones in the supine position, with the legs against the wall at a 90-degree angle in parallel alignment.

>> Move close into the wall and lengthen the heels away from your sit bones. Make sure your sit bones are not lifted toward the ceiling. You don't need to have your buttocks touching the wall. Keep the pelvis in neutral alignment.

>> Press the heels lightly into the wall and slowly open the legs sideways. Keep the legs parallel.

>> Hold for ten slow breaths or up to 60 seconds. You should feel a stretch along the inside thighs.

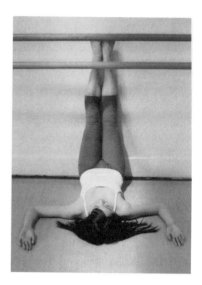

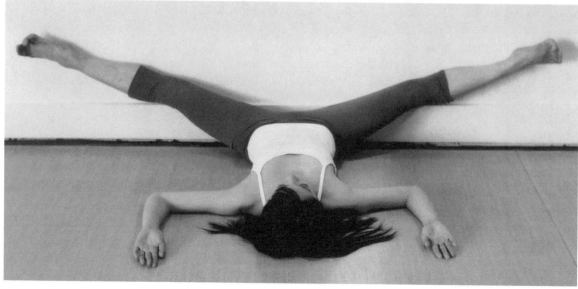

INSIDE THIGH STRETCH ON THE WALL IN OUTWARD ROTATION »

Explore the different sensations between the parallel and outward rotated stretches.

>> Align the bones in the supine position with the legs against the wall at a 90-degree angle in a slightly outward rotation.

>> Move close into the wall and lengthen the heels away from your sit bones. You don't need to have your buttocks touching the wall. Keep the pelvis in neutral alignment. Make sure the sit bones are not lifted toward the ceiling.

>> Press the heels lightly into the wall and slowly open the legs sideways. Keep the legs in slight outward rotation.

>> Hold for ten slow breaths or up to 60 seconds. You should feel a stretch along the inside thighs and hamstrings.

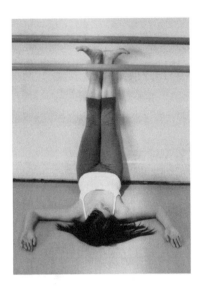

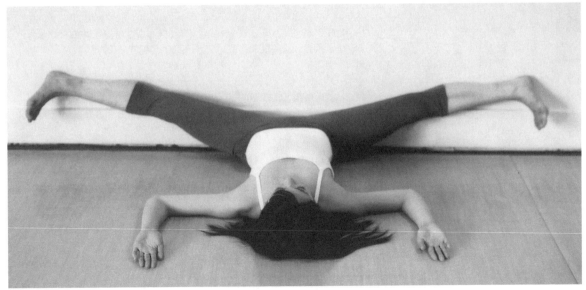

BEGINNER HAMSTRING STRETCH, STANDING LOW »

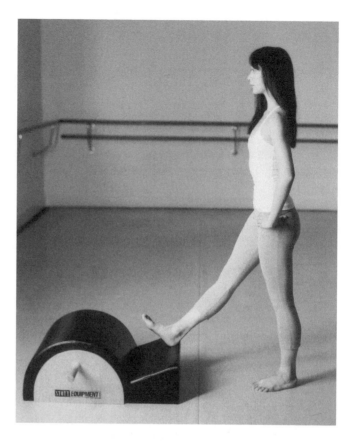

Keep your pelvis, lower back and hips healthy with daily hamstring stretches, especially if you spend much of your working day sitting.

» Align the bones in the standing position, with your hands on your hips or resting on a chair or table of suitable height to help you balance.

» Extend your right leg forward in line with your sit bone in parallel alignment. Rest your heel on low-lying equipment, such as a low stool or a block. Keep the ankle soft as you flex your foot. Be careful not to press the back of the extended knee down to the floor.

» Do not twist your hips by allowing the right hip to come forward.

» Hinge your body slightly forward from the hips, without swinging the pelvis or the standing leg backward.

» Maintain a neutral spine. Do not hunch over. Lengthen the tailbone and the crown of the head away from each other. You should feel a gentle stretch through the hamstring at the back of the upper leg.

» Hold for ten breaths or 60 seconds before moving to the other side.

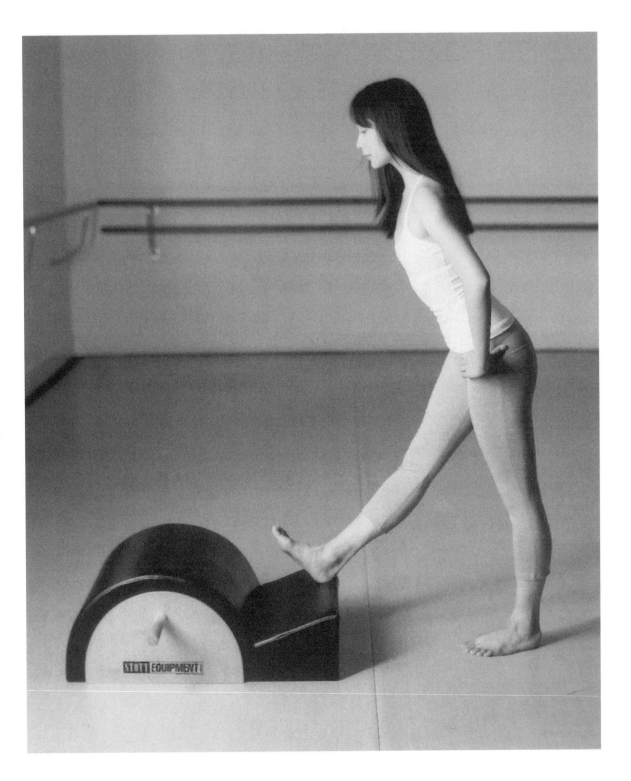

INTERMEDIATE HAMSTRING STRETCH, KNEELING >>

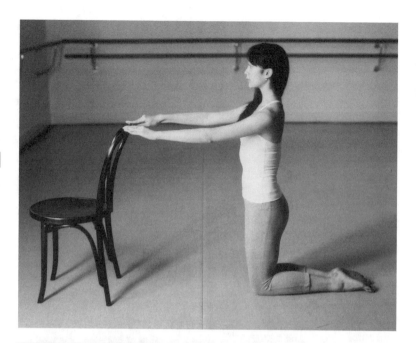

>> Kneel upright behind the back of a chair, about an arm's length away. Place your hands on the back of the chair. Find a neutral spinal alignment.

>> Extend your right leg forward in line with your sit bone in parallel alignment, resting your heel on the floor with a slightly flexed foot. Be careful not to press the back of the extended knee down to the floor.

>> Do not twist your hips by allowing the right hip to come forward.

>> Hinge your body slightly forward from the hips without swinging the pelvis or the kneeling leg backward. Bend your elbows slightly as your body moves forward.

>> Maintain a neutral spine. Do not hunch over. Hold for ten breaths or 60 seconds before moving to the other side.

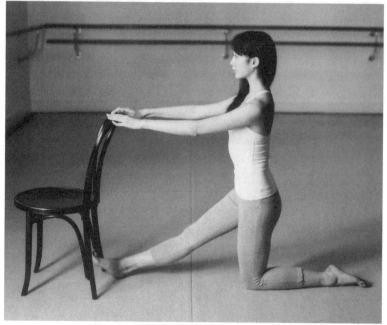

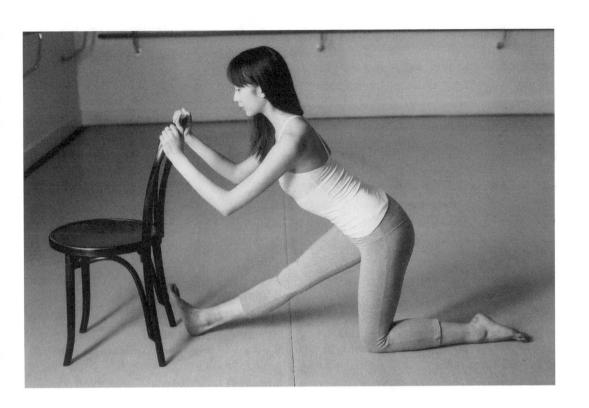

ADVANCED HAMSTRING
STRETCH, STANDING HIGH ⟩⟩

Once you gain confidence with this stretch you can perform it in the same way as the "beginner hamstring stretch" but with the extended leg on a higher piece of equipment, such as a chair or bench, depending on your flexibility. Remember to maintain neutral pelvic alignment and don't work into pain.

BEGINNER ILIOPSOAS, KNEELING »

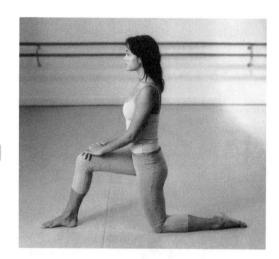

This is also a good daily rebalancing stretch to assist with general mobility if you sit a great deal during the day.

>> Kneel upright and find a neutral spinal alignment. You might like to hold on to the back of a chair for extra support.

>> Take the right leg forward, making a 90-degree angle.

>> Gently move the tailbone underneath you toward the right foot and try to make the shape of a small C curve with the lower back.

>> You should feel a stretch through the front of your left hip and up into your torso.

>> Hold the stretch for five breaths and repeat on the other side.

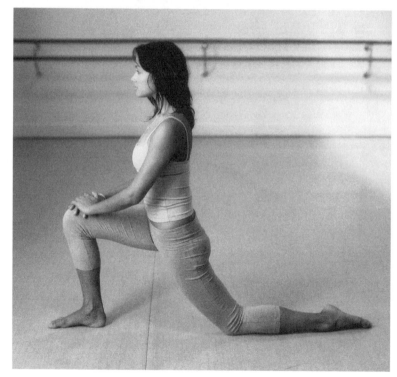

ADVANCED ILIOPSOAS, LUNGING »

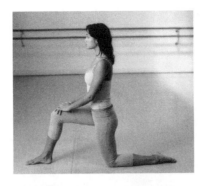

>> Kneel upright and find a neutral spinal alignment. You might like to hold on to the back of a chair for extra support.

>> Take the right leg forward, making a 90-degree angle.

>> Gently move the tailbone underneath you toward the right foot and try to make the shape of a small C curve with the lower back (lumbar).

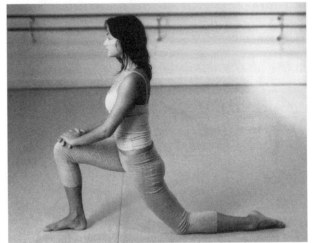

>> Maintaining the C curve in the lower back, tuck the toes of the left foot under and take the left knee from the floor, reaching the left heel away from the left sit bone. Move as far as is comfortable, keeping the hips level, with a sense of reach in the back leg. Keep your front knee facing straight ahead and feel the front foot melting into the ground.

>> Hold for up to five breaths and repeat on the other side.

>> As you gain confidence with this stretch you can let go of the chair and place your hands on your knee or on top of your head.

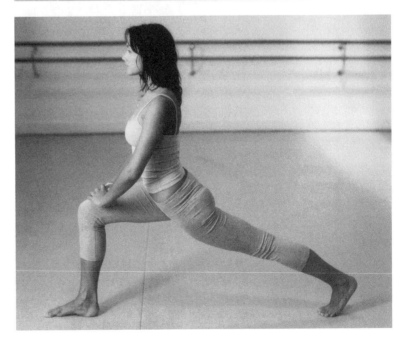

STANDING THIGH
STRETCH »

» Align your bones in the standing position, with your hands placed on the back of a chair for support.

» Bend your right knee and take hold of the top arch of your foot with your right hand, bringing your foot toward the buttocks, not necessarily touching. Don't over-compress the knee joint. You shouldn't feel discomfort behind the knee joint or a pulling sensation in the knee cap.

» Keep the legs parallel and try to keep the knees touching. Maintain spinal and pelvic alignment.

» Hold for ten slow breaths or 60 seconds and repeat with the other leg.

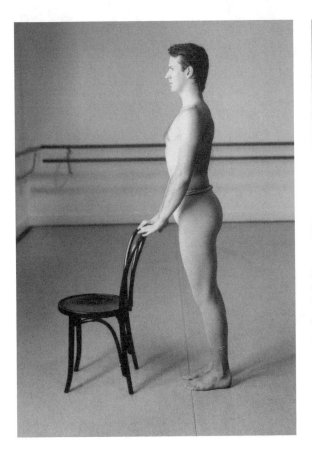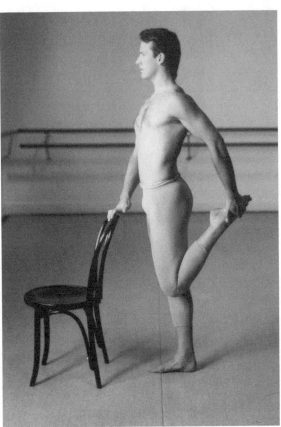

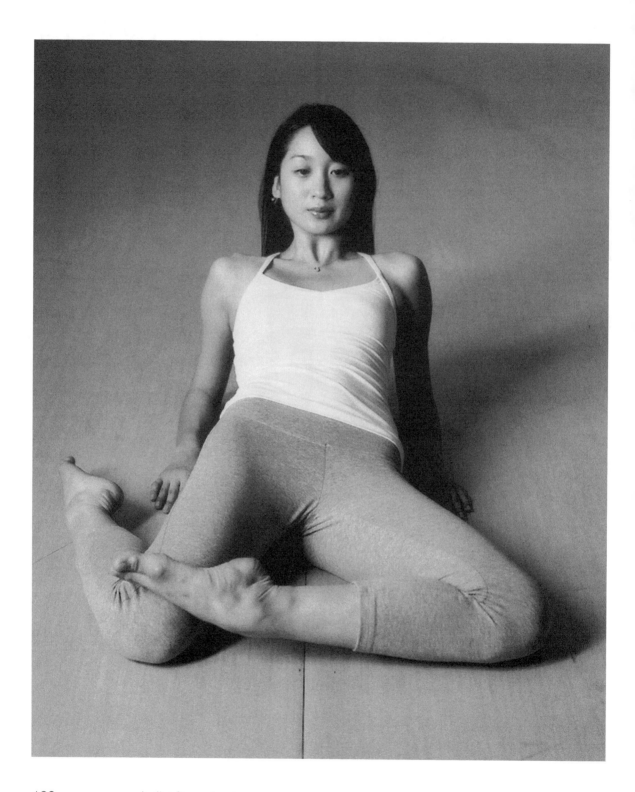

« ballet-fit workout »

ADVANCED
THIGH STRETCH »

» Align your bones in the sitting
position with your legs extended
in front of you.

» Lean your body to the left and
bring the right foot along the
floor toward the buttocks.

» Carefully bend the left knee and
place the heel on top of the
right knee.

» Slide your sit bones away from
the floor, toward the ceiling,
making a small C in the
lower back.

» Rest back on your elbows.

» Hold the stretch for ten breaths
or 60 seconds.

» Turn toward the left and slowly
unfold the left leg to come out
of the position safely.

» Repeat on the other side.

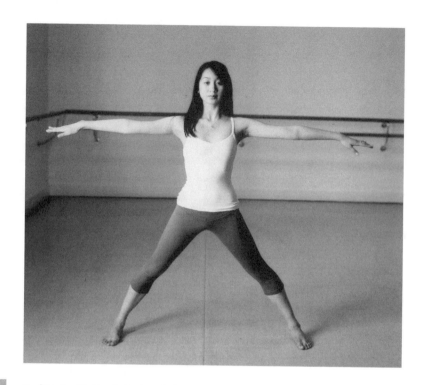

ADVANCED
BACK AND LEG
STRETCH »

This brings the stretch to the back and inside legs and a lovely sense of release through the spine.

» Stand with the feet placed about a leg's length apart in parallel alignment with toes pointing forward. Reach the arms sideways, with palms facing toward the floor.

» Drop your head and roll down through the spine, articulating each vertebra until your hands reach the floor. Place the hands directly under the shoulders to begin with, for initial stability. Your elbows should point toward the back wall.

» If your hamstring range is limited, try resting your hands on a low table or a block.

» Lengthen the spine toward the floor and the sit bones up toward the ceiling. Don't swing back on the legs.

» Move the weight of the body over the front of each ankle and feel the weight distributed through the three points of each foot.

» Stay here for ten breaths.

» If you want a more intense stretch, walk your hands through the legs, keeping your elbows pointing toward the back wall.

» Slowly reverse the movements to recover.

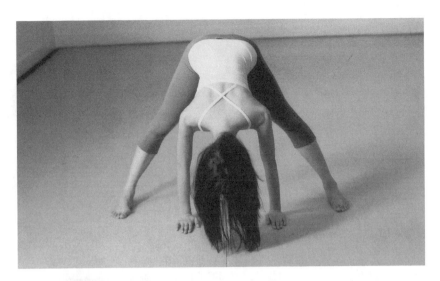

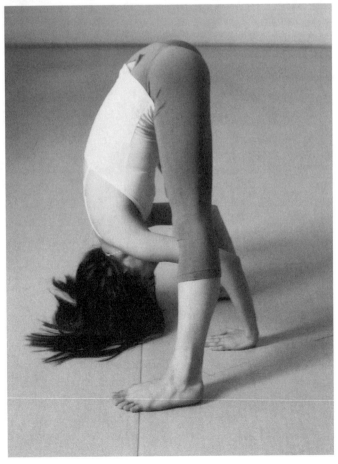

ROLL DOWN
AND WALK OUT 》》

Keep this stretch slow and even in its movements and increase the speed and add it to a warm-up as a spinal mobilizer.

>> Align your bones in the standing position.

>> Keeping your center of gravity over the front of the ankles, take your chin down toward your throat and begin to roll down through the spine. Keep the crown of your head falling toward your feet and try not to hinge forward at the hips or lower back.

>> Articulate each vertebra as you move through the spine until your hands touch the floor. If necessary your legs can softly bend here to place your hands on the floor and then work toward gently stretching the legs.

>> Allow the elbows to bend and continue until the crown of your head is as close to the floor as possible. You can soften your knees slightly to ease any tightness at the back of the legs.

>> Walk the hands forward into a wide V or as far as the stretch feels comfortable. To make sure the spine alignment stays neutral, drop your head down in line with the spine. Encourage the tailbone toward the ceiling.

>> Keep your hands one shoulder's width apart, with the palms flat and fingers wide. Keep the sit bones pointing toward the ceiling.

>> Each time you do the exercise, think of lengthening the back of the leg by directing the sit bones to the ceiling and the heels toward the floor to encourage a stretch the back the legs and lumbar spine. Over time your flexibility will improve.

>> Slowly reverse all the movements to return to the standing position.

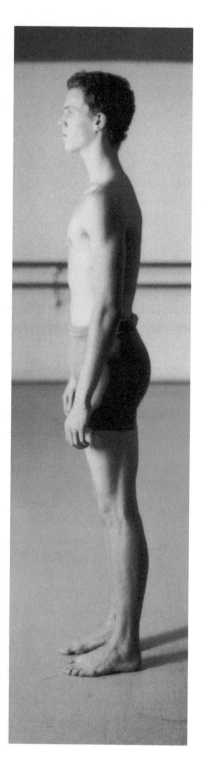

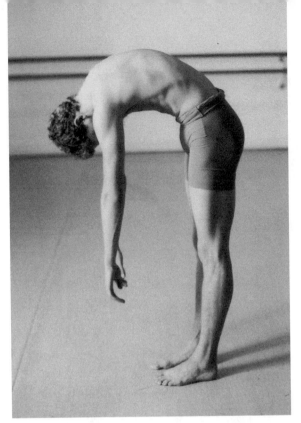

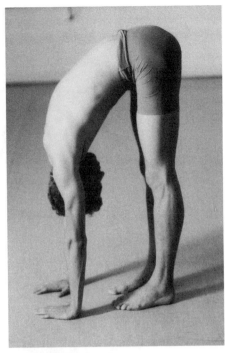

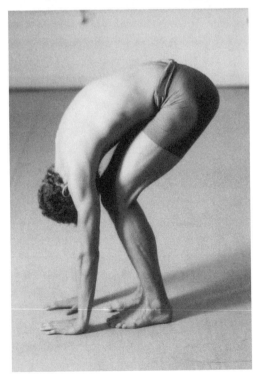

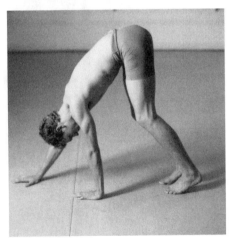

BIG V PRESS >>

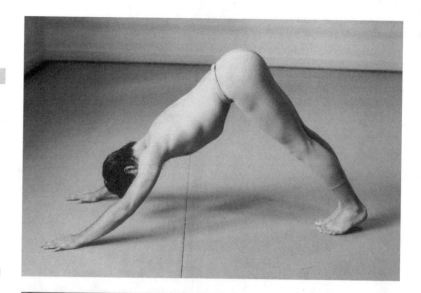

The purpose of this stretch is to work the whole length of the back of the body, from the shoulders to the Achilles, through a lengthening process. It also stimulates the iliopsoas and broadens the shoulders and back.

>> Do the roll down and walk out on page 196 until you have walked out to a wide inverted V shape.

>> Send your sit bones to the ceiling and work your heels toward the floor.

>> Lengthen the spine and reach the head away from the tailbone.

>> Hold for up to ten breaths or 60 seconds.

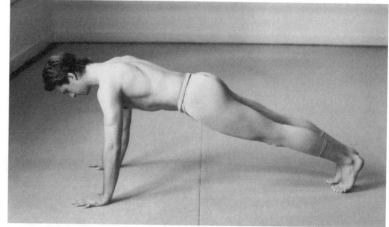

>> Lower your body into a push-up position. Alternatively, once you have made the wide V position you can bend your knees and move toward the floor into the "child's pose" on page 171.

>> Continue to lower your body all the way to the floor.

>> Then press up. Fold at the hips and return to the V shape. Repeat this up to five times and hold each V shape for ten breaths.

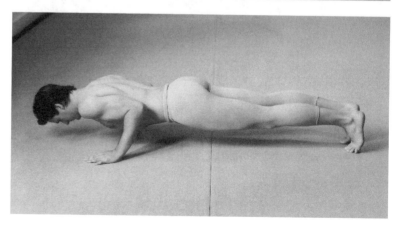

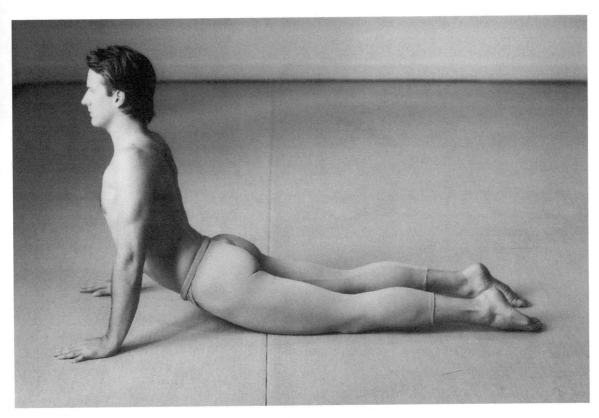

SPHINX »

Try to focus on the sternum reaching forward. Use your eyes to focus your energy and keep the spine lengthening.

» Align your bones in the prone position, with your hands by your shoulders and elbows bent. Rest your forehead on the floor.

» Lengthen the sternum forward along the floor and up toward the ceiling.

» Straighten the arms slowly and lengthen the spine out of the lower lumbar to curve the back. Repeat five times or hold for up to five breaths. For a modified version keep the hands and elbows on the floor. Do not straighten the arms before returning to the floor.

» Slowly reverse the action to return to the supine position.

» You can then bend the knees and fold back into the "child's pose" on page 171.

ATTENTION TO DETAIL *If you feel any discomfort in the lower lumbar, stop and work on the "diamond press" exercise on page 98.*

LUNGING
CALF STRETCH »

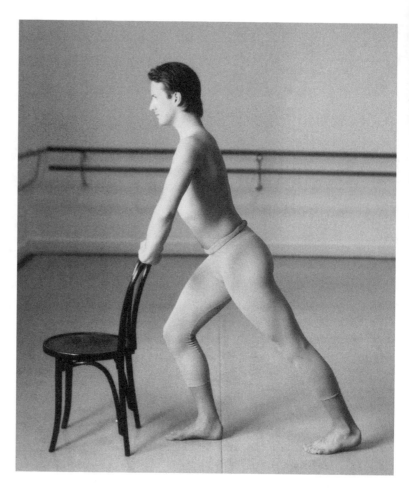

This exercise can also be done using a wall for support.

>> Align your bones in the standing position and stand one step away from the back of a chair.

>> Step your right foot forward, bending your knee, and place your hands on the chair. Allow the heel of your left leg to release off the floor.

>> Keep both feet parallel, with toes pointing forward.

>> Keep the spine long and neutral.

>> To begin the stretch, reach the heel of the left leg toward the floor and encourage your weight forward over the front leg.

>> Press your weight through the big toe or the small toe of the back foot to move the stretch into a different area of the calf muscle.

>> Sustain the stretch for ten breaths.

>> Repeat on the other side.

KNEELING ACHILLES STRETCH »

A gentle mobilizing stretch for the Achilles.

» Kneeling on the right knee, place the ends of the toes of the left foot in line with the right knee, maintaining parallel alignment.

» Rest back on your right heel, keeping the left heel on the floor. Fold your arms over the top of the left knee.

» Take your body weight forward toward the left knee and let the weight of the chest move the knee forward and toward the floor. The left heel will most likely come off the floor.

» Feel the opposing pull of falling forward to the left knee as the left heel reaches to the floor.

» Hold for ten breaths, then repeat on the other side.

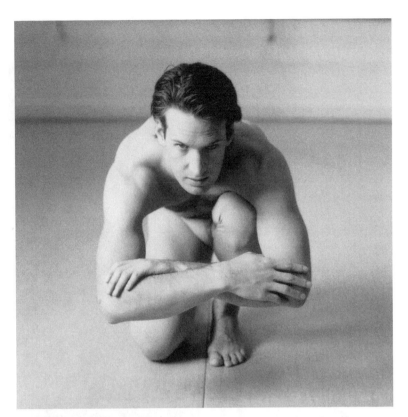

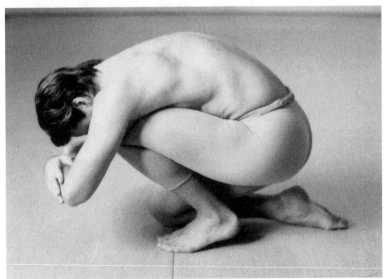

WALKING OVER
A STICK >>

This exercise helps to release tension from the bottom of your feet.

>> Align your bones in the standing position.

>> Step the balls of your feet onto a stick or thin broom handle and rest for a short time. Try to relax your weight into the stick.

>> Gently transfer the weight from one foot to the other.

>> Continue to walk your feet across the stick in about half-inch increments, resting at each point and gently transferring the weight from one foot to the other, until you have walked all the way over the stick.

>> Take your time. The whole process can take more than 60 seconds but not longer than 5 minutes.

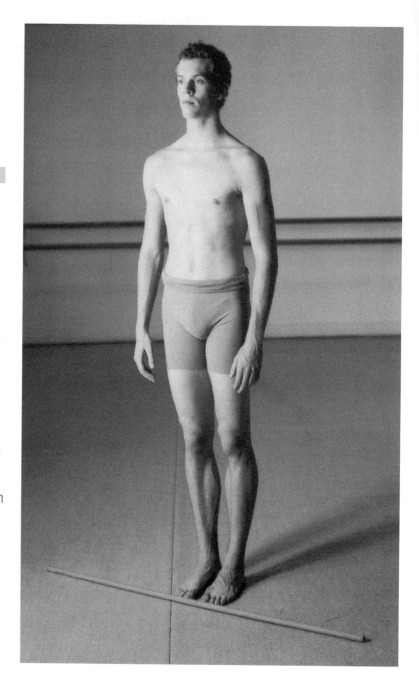

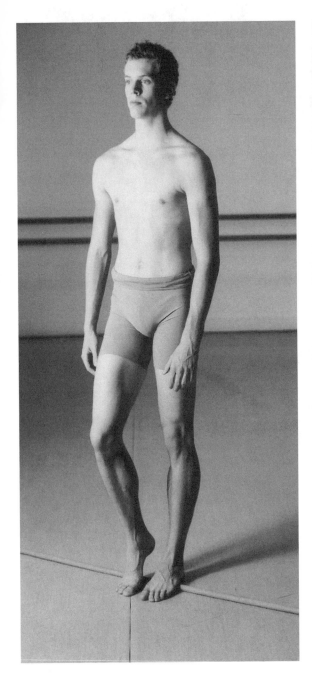

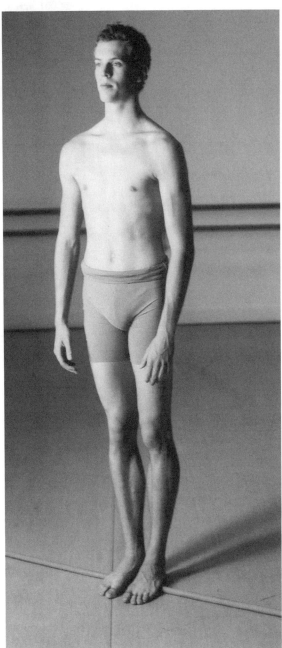

« lengthen and release »   203

WORKING ON THE WOBBLE-BOARD »

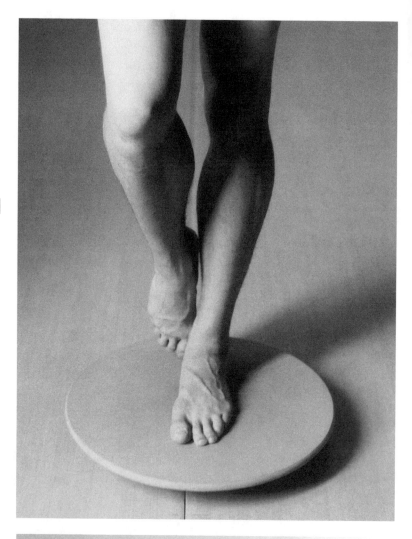

A wobble-board is a circular balancing board with a metallic half-sphere attached under-neath. You may have seen one in a gym or when visiting a physical therapist's office.

Wobble-boards are often used by dancers to fine-tune their kinetic awareness. These boards highlight alignment and work the deep stabilizers more intensely, due to the re-balancing required by being on an unstable base. If you have the chance to try out a wobble-board, remember that the more tension you hold, the harder it will be to balance. Relax, align the bones, fall off and get back on. If you persevere you will improve your balance and develop a sense of good alignment.

Things you can do on a wobble-board include:

» Finding your alignment in the standing position on two legs.

» Finding your alignment in the standing position on one leg.

» Spinal waves, standing.

» Arm float series, standing.

» Spinal twist, standing.

» Add anything adventurous, even rising to the toes, and don't worry about falling off.

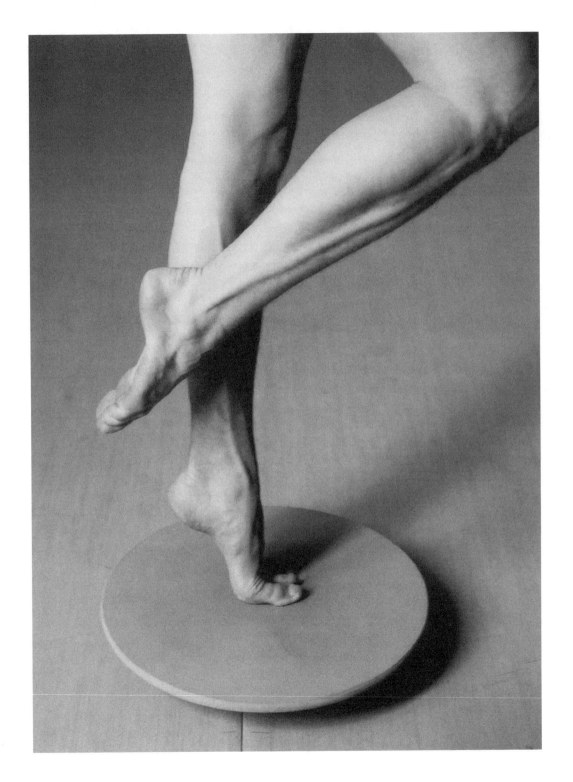

The authors

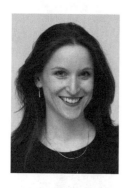

>> Megan Connelly

As a professional dancer, Megan joined The Australian Ballet in 1991 under the direction of Maina Gielgud and was later invited to join the artistic staff as Assistant to the Ballet Staff.

Since leaving the company in 1995 Megan has pursued a teaching career, specializing in training students for a professional career in dance. In 1999 Megan toured to Germany as Ballet Mistress for the *Year 2000 Project*. Her guest teaching engagements include schools and companies in Australia and Europe, and she has also performed with Opera Australia and as an independent artist.

After receiving an Award of Excellence in Business Computing she returned to The Australian Ballet in 2001 under the direction of David McAllister as Personal Assistant to the Artistic Director. In addition to her administrative tasks she also teaches company class and works with the dancers, medical team and ballet staff in the area of coaching and rehabilitation.

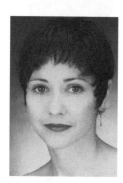

>> Paula Baird-Colt

Paula Baird-Colt danced with West Australian Ballet from 1983 to 1987, when she joined The Australian Ballet. She was promoted to Coryphée in 1990 and to Soloist in 1995. In 1993 she received a Green Room Award for Best Female Dancer in a Supporting Role in *Sand Siren*.

Paula has performed in many productions with The Australian Ballet including major roles in *Of Blessed Memory, Catalyst, Jardí Tancat, Sinfonietta, In the Upper Room,* Tatiana in *Onegin,* Suzuki in *Madame Butterfly* and the Jealous Sister in *Las Hermanas*. Other works included *Beyond Bach, In the Middle, Somewhat Elevated, Red Earth* and *The Deep End*.

In 2000 Paula left The Australian Ballet and in 2002 became a certified Pilates Instructor. She currently teaches Body Conditioning and Stretching for The Australian Ballet School and The Australian Ballet.

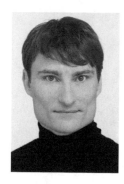

>> David McAllister
Artistic Director

A graduate of The Australian Ballet School, Perth-born David McAllister began his training with Evelyn Hodgkinson and joined The Australian Ballet in 1983. He was promoted to Senior Artist in 1986 and to Principal Artist in January 1989.

His principal roles have included those in *Onegin, Romeo and Juliet, La Fille Mal Gardée, The Sleeping Beauty, Don Quixote, The Sentimental Bloke, Coppélia, Manon, La Sylphide, Sinfonietta* and *Stepping Stones*.

In 1985 he won a Bronze Medal at the Fifth International Ballet Competition in Moscow and the same year won the Oceanic Equity Arts Award for Young Achievers in Perth. As a result of the Moscow Competition he was invited to return to the USSR as a guest artist and made numerous appearances with the Bolshoi Ballet, the Kirov Ballet, the Georgian State Ballet and other companies in *Don Quixote*, in *Giselle* and in gala performances.

David McAllister danced for the final time in *Giselle* on 24 March 2001 at the Sydney Opera House and became Artistic Director of The Australian Ballet in July 2001. He was awarded a Member of the Order of Australia in the 2004 Australia Day Honors List.

The dancers

>> Adam Bull
Coryphée

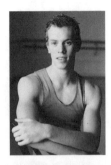

Adam graduated from The Australian Ballet School in 2001 with honors and joined The Australian Ballet in 2002. He has performed in *Spartacus*, *Beyond 40*, Graeme Murphy's *Swan Lake* and the world premieres of Adrian Burnett's *Subtle Sequence of Revelation* and Meryl Tankard's *Wild Swans*. He has also performed principal and soloist roles in *The Three Musketeers* and *Symphony in C* and soloist roles in the Australian premiere of *Agon*. Adam performed in Elizabeth Hill's *Link* and Paulina Quinteros' *Awakening* and *Venetian Summer* as part of the inaugural "bodytorque" season.

>> Natalie Decorte
Corps de Ballet

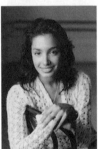

Natalie joined The Australian Ballet School in 1997 and completed her training at The Royal Ballet School in London. After dancing with The Royal Ballet for five years, she joined The Australian Ballet in July 2003. She has appeared in productions of *Molto Vivace*, *Swan Lake*, *The Three Musketeers* and *Symphony in C*.

>> Joshua Horner

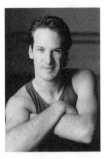

Joshua Horner joined The Australian Ballet in 1999. He performed roles in *Dark Lullaby*, *X*, *Por vos Muero*, *In the Upper Room*, Hilarion in *Giselle* and *Tivoli*. In 2002 he was nominated for a Helpmann Award for his role in *Tivoli*. In July 2004 Joshua left The Australian Ballet to pursue a career in musical theater.

>> Natasha Kusen
Corps de Ballet

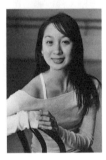

In 2001 Natasha won a scholarship at the Prix de Lausanne to study at The Royal Ballet School in London. She joined The Australian Ballet in 2003 and has since performed in *Serenade*, *Symphony in C*, *Swan Lake* and Christopher Wheeldon's *Continuum©*.

» Acknowledgments

» The Australian Ballet

David McAllister
Megan Connelly
Paula Baird-Colt
Adam Bull
Natalie Decorte
Joshua Horner
Natasha Kusen
Noelle Shader
Nicolette Fraillon
Richard Evans
Patrick McIntyre
Yvonne Gates
Helen McCormack

ballet-fit workout is approved by The Australian Ballet's Medical Team

» ABC Books

Jill Brown
Jody Lee
Nanette Backhouse

» Photography

Pierre Baroni
Portraits Jeff Busby and Branco Gaica

» Special thanks

to **BODY** clothing